Gender, Eating Disorders, and Graphic Medicine

W0113686

Developing an understanding of eating diso   s beyond the biological/
medical framework has become a necessit   esent times, especially
when eating disorders are swiftly spreading   roots across the world.
In view of the multidimensional etiology of eating disorders, there are
increased efforts towards understanding its phenomenological, cultural,
and other related non-medical aspects, and *Gender, Eating Disorders,
and Graphic Medicine* leaps past the prevalent notions on eating disorder, and contributes to the developing corpus of affective knowledge on
eating disorders among women through comics and graphic medicine.
Taking cues from select graphic narratives on eating disorders, this book
attempts to posit graphic medicine as one of the most befitting modes
of life writing. This book is distinctive in that it is an attempt not only
to explore the multi-dimensional etiology of eating disorders in women
using graphic medicine narratives but also to understand how graphic
medicine humanizes eating disorders by offering a unique ingress into
women's phenomenological experience of eating disorders.

Anu Mary Peter was a Jawaharlal Nehru doctoral research fellow in the
Department of Humanities and Social Sciences at the National Institute
of Technology, Trichy (India). She is currently an independent health humanities researcher. Her research articles have appeared in various Web
of Science/Scopus indexed journals such as *Health: An International Journal for Social Study of Health, Illness and Medicine, Journal of Graphic
Novels and Comics*, and *INKS: The Journal of the Comics Studies Society*,
among others. She is the author of a collection of poems titled *My Impossible Highway* (2015).

Sathyaraj Venkatesan is an Associate Professor of English, Department of
Humanities and Social Sciences, National Institute of Technology, Trichy
(India). His research concentrates on illness narratives, graphic medicine,
and literature and medicine. He is the author of four books and more than
eighty research articles. His most recent volume of co-edited essays is
titled *The Idea and Practice of Reading* (2018).

Gender, Eating Disorders, and Graphic Medicine

**Anu Mary Peter
and Sathyaraj Venkatesan**

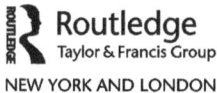

Routledge
Taylor & Francis Group

NEW YORK AND LONDON

First published 2021
by Routledge
52 Vanderbilt Avenue, New York, NY 10017

and by Routledge
2 Park Square, Milton Park, Abingdon, Oxon, OX14 4RN

Routledge is an imprint of the Taylor & Francis Group, an informa business

© 2021 Taylor & Francis

The right of Anu Mary Peter and Sathyaraj Venkatesan
to be identified as authors of this work has been asserted
by them in accordance with sections 77 and 78 of the
Copyright, Designs and Patents Act 1988.

All rights reserved. No part of this book may be reprinted
or reproduced or utilised in any form or by any electronic,
mechanical, or other means, now known or hereafter
invented, including photocopying and recording, or in
any information storage or retrieval system, without
permission in writing from the publishers.

Trademark notice: Product or corporate names may
be trademarks or registered trademarks, and are used
only for identification and explanation without intent to
infringe.

Library of Congress Cataloging-in-Publication Data
A catalog record for this title has been requested

ISBN: 978-0-367-44300-9 (hbk)
ISBN: 978-0-367-54085-2 (pbk)
ISBN: 978-1-003-08756-4 (ebk)

Typeset in Times New Roman
by codeMantra

Contents

Introduction   1
Eating Disorders, Biocultures, and Graphic Medicine 2
Why Graphic Medicine? 3
Overview of the Book 5

1   A Prologue to Graphic Medicine   8
Medical Humanities: Towards the Humanization of
  Medical Science 8
Narrative Medicine: Understanding the Ordeals of Illness 9
Spectacles of Suffering: Representation of Illness
  across Media 10
Comics Medium and Healthcare 11
Comics, Women, and the Counterculture 12
Graphic Medicine: Definition and Scope 13
Conclusion 14

2   Clinical Evolution of Eating Disorders and the
Rise of the Biocultures   17
Chronicles of Starvation: A Cultural History of
  Eating Disorders 18
The Middle Ages: Fasting Saints and Miracle Maidens 18
From Miracle to Madness and Hysteria 19
Eating Disorders: A Medical Introduction 21
  Anorexia Nervosa 22
  Bulimia Nervosa 22
  Binge Eating and EDNOS 23
Pitfalls in the Popular Explanatory Models of Eating
  Disorders 23

The Biocultural Model   25
Tracing the Footprints of Culture in Science   26
Graphic Medicine and the Biocultures   29
Conclusion   29

3   **Warped Femininities: Understanding the Corporeal**
     Nexus of Anorexia and Culture   33
     The Ideal Female Body as a Cultural Construct   34
     Anorexia Nervosa: A Biocultural Approach   36
     "At That Time, Nobody Considered It": Anorexia and
          Familial Pressure   38
          Guilt   40
          Punishment   42
     "Neil! You Look Like a Man!": Body Shaming and
          Anorexia   43
     "As Long as I'm Thin . . . I'll Be Invincible": Media
          and Thinspiration   47
     Conclusion   51
     Acknowledgment   52

4   **Subjective Incarnations of Anorexia: Creative**
     Metaphors and Graphic Externalization   56
     Comics, Metaphors, and Externalization   57
     Graphic Medicine and the Iconography of Illness   59
     "I'm Tyranny, Your Other Self": The Metaphor of
          Self-Oppression   60
     "My Ed—So Big and STRONG": Relationship
          Metaphors in Anorexia Narratives   64
     Dark Clouds of Despair: The Metaphor of Pervasiveness   66
     Epitomizing the Indefinable: The Power of
          Comics Medium   68
     Conclusion   70
     Acknowledgment   72

5   **From Abjection to Anorexia: Eating Disorders and the**
     Horrors of the Female Body   75
     Feminist Perspectives on Eating Disorders   76
     Abjection: Origin, and Popular Definitions   77

Abjection and Anorexia: Theoretical Interventions of
    Megan Warin 79
"*I Feel Disgusting*": *Menstruation and Abjection in*
    Lighter Than My Shadow *82*
"*I Hate This. I Hate Me*": *Menstruation and*
    Abjection in Tyranny *87*
"*I'm Disgusting*": *Self-Disgust and Sexual Abuse* 90
Conclusion 94

**Conclusion: Towards an Alternative Understanding
of Eating Disorders**   98

Acknowledgments   104

Index   107

Introduction

In June of 2019, an article appeared in *The Guardian* offering a significant disclosure about the failure of the existing medical system in fathoming the etiology and treatment procedures of eating disorders adequately. Provocatively titled as 'Doctors' Failings on Eating Disorders are Costing Lives,' the article reiterates the observations from the report of the Parliamentary Select Committee, and states: "the [l]ack of understanding of eating disorders among doctors is resulting in too many avoidable deaths, with medical staff receiving too little training" (Davies). Although eating disorders have received medical attention at least since the seventeenth century, its rate of incidence is rapidly increasing. Developing a renewed understanding of eating disorders beyond the biological/medical framework has become a necessity in present times, especially when eating disorders are swiftly spreading deep roots across the world. Therefore, to reconfigure the popular perception of eating disorders, efforts must be taken to understand the phenomenological, cultural, and other related non-medical aspects of the illness condition.

As Cynthia Bulik, the founding director of the Center of Excellence for Eating Disorders at the University of North Carolina at Chapel Hill, exhorts, "[w]e must change how every physician and therapist learns about eating disorders and erase past false theories and hypotheses" by acknowledging the instrumental role of socio-cultural and environmental factors (Lewis). Interestingly, it is less challenging to attain a holistic understanding of the various causes of eating disorders using the biocultural theory, which productively combines the medical and cultural factors. In view of the "multifactorial perspective, there has been an increased movement towards understanding the emotional complexity of eating disorders" and this book contributes to the developing corpus of phenomenological knowledge on eating disorders among women through graphic medicine (Foye et al. 322). Unlike other modes of life writing, comics facilitates visual thinking and verbo-visual expression of experiences. The ability of graphic medicine "to incorporate and integrate the visual equally alongside the verbal, facilitate and offer the capacity for more whole ways of expression and representation" (Sousanis 1) makes it suitable for the narration of experiences that are too complex to be communicated verbally.

Eating Disorders, Biocultures, and Graphic Medicine

Followed by the clinical classification of anorexia in the nineteenth century as an illness condition seen among women, various explanatory models such as the biomedical model, psychological model, cultural model, psycho-social model, and feminist model emerged. However, each model defined eating disorders from specific perspectives of medicine and psychiatry, and therefore, all of them offered incomplete explanations for the rise of eating disorders in women. Further, all of them failed in explaining the fundamental cause for the prevalence of eating disorders among women, especially in non-western societies. For a long time, it remained an underexplored fact that eating disorders can be caused as a result of a combination of biological, cultural, and psychological factors. Interestingly, when all other models failed to offer a convincing theoretical explanation for the eating disorder conundrum, the biocultures model could adequately theorize the causes of the high incidence rate of eating disorders among women by factoring its biological as well as cultural roots.

The biocultural model was formulated by Lennard J. Davis and David B. Morris using George Engel's biopsychosocial model of illness. Biocultures offers a holistic method to investigate eating disorders, especially anorexia nervosa, by yoking together the biomedical model and the cultural model of eating disorders. The biocultural model underlines the multidimensional etiology of eating disorders and critiques the constricted approach that biomedicine has towards the causes of eating disorders. Similarly, the biocultural model, by bringing together medicine and culture, expands the prospects of eating disorder research beyond biology and psychiatry.

While comics and medicine were culturally linked long before the emergence of graphic medicine, it was in the latter half of the twentieth century that comics flourished beyond the realms of entertainment as a medium fit for auto/biographical narrations

(Meskin and Cook xxiv). Accordingly, comics have always played a central role in the cultural representation of the female body in crisis. Especially, comics medium was deployed during the underground comix era as one of the most popular methods to discuss female concerns about body, sexuality. Although many graphic illness memoirs published before 2007 evince the quintessential qualities of graphic medicine—for instance, Justin Green's *Binky Brown Meets the Holy Virgin Mary* (1972), Al Davison's *The Spiral Cage* (1990), and Harvey Pekar and Joyce Brabner's *Our Cancer Year* (1994)—it was with the formulation of the graphic medicine collective in 2007 that graphic narratives of illness experiences gained an identity of their own. In Gesine Wegner's words, the success of graphic novels is "indicative of a general graphic memoir boom in the twenty-first century" and graphic narratives have become "the fastest growing category within the [American] literary market (Fingeroth vii)" (60). Wegner further states that the advancement of graphic pathography is due to "the overall popularity of autobiographical comics at the beginning of the twenty-first century, and because the genre seems to further satisfy an existing interest in illness and disability memoirs" (4).

The term graphic medicine was coined by Ian Williams, a British physician in 2007, during the commencement of the website-*graphicmedicine.org*. Followed by the formulation of the online platform, notable academicians and healthcare practitioners such as M. K. Czerwiec, Michael J. Green, Kimberly R. Myers, Susan M. Squier, and Scott T. Smith joined the graphic medicine core team. In 2010, when Green and Myers published an article titled "Graphic Medicine: Use of Comics in Medical Education and Patient Care" in *BMJ*, graphic medicine started garnering more popularity as a field of study. Today, as a subset of comics, graphic medicine offers a narrative space for the marginalized community of sufferers, which comprises of patients, caregivers, and healthcare providers, to communicate their subjective experiential truths.

Why Graphic Medicine?

While a barrage of literary autobiographies on eating disorders in women have emerged since 1978, not many have been successful in pushing beyond the philanthropic and cathartic imperatives of autobiographical writing. When most of the available memoirs remain guide books on treatment and diet plans with scant glimpses of affective realities, graphic medicine narratives delineate that eating disorders are caused by a plethora of experiences that are often too traumatic to be verbalized. Beyond the traditionally set imperatives and age-old promises of the autobiography as a genre, autopathographies (autobiographical comics on illness experiences) offer a nuanced way for marginalized sufferers to reshuffle the prevailing notions and misconceptions of illness, suffering, and recovery. The distinctive capacity to easily establish a visual connection helps artists to make the reader experience what they have gone through without losing much of its intensity during translation. Essentially, the infinite representational potential of comics medium to accurately and credibly represent marginalized subjectivity helps to add uniquely subjective labyrinths to universal experiences of illnesses.

Compared to the popular portrayals of eating disorders in verbal narratives or movies, graphic medicine narratives deal with diverse perspectives on the biocultural and feminine experiences of eating disorders that are hitherto underexplored. Unfortunately, there is no significant scholarship on how verbo-visual narratives or graphic memoirs facilitate a holistic understanding of the etiology and repercussions of eating disorders on women. Apart from a handful of research articles, such as Ian Williams' "Autography as Auto-Therapy: Psychic Pain and the Graphic Memoir" (2011), Michelle N. Huang's "Review of Katie Green's *Lighter Than My Shadow*" (2014), and unpublished articles, such as "A Close Analysis of Clinical Framings of Anorexia Nervosa in *Lighter Than My Shadow*" and "Drawing Unspeakable Trauma: Representations of the Abject in Katie Green's *Lighter Than My Shadow*" by Emma Louise Pudge, Karen McFayden's "Art, Alienation, and Assumed Aesthetics in Katie Green's *Lighter Than My Shadow*" (2016), and Miroslav Kupka's Bachelor Thesis titled "Psychopathological Phenomena in Karrie Fransman's Graphic Novel *The House that Groaned*," there are no substantial research works available on graphic medicine narratives and eating disorders.

Considering the minimal focus that eating disorder narratives have received in comics studies, this book aims to add to the evolving body of research on graphic medicine and eating disorders by close reading seven graphic narratives: Nadia Shivack's *Inside Out: Portrait of an Eating Disorder* (2007), Carol Lay's *The Big Skinny: How I Changed My Fattitude* (2008), Lesley Fairfield's *Tyranny* (2009), Ludovic Debeurme's *Lucille* (2011), Karrie Fransman's *The House That Groaned* (2012), Katie Green's *Lighter Than My Shadow* (2013), and *Ink in Water: An Illustrated Memoir (Or, How I Kicked Anorexia's Ass and Embraced Body Positivity)* by Lacy J. Davis and

Jim Kettner (2016). Departing from the popular descriptions of eating disorders, these graphic narratives on women's eating disorder experiences facilitate an interface between disordered eating and the agony caused by a plethora of biocultural factors.

Fundamentally, by close reading seven graphic narratives, this book aims to analyze: (1) various ways in which women experience their bodies as abject, disgusting, and shameful due to its non-conformity with the prevalent body ideals; (2) how women resort to starvation or binge as an aftermath of the derailed relationship with their bodies; and (3) how the emotional scars from various traumatic and shameful incidents further precipitate the aversion to their body and self, eventually leading to eating disorders. Taking cues from select graphic narratives, and by drawing theoretical insights from Joan Jacob Brumberg, Susan Bordo, Lennard J. Davis, David B. Morris, Megan Warin, Elizabeth El Refaie, and other theoreticians, this book aims to demonstrate how a gendered biocultural analysis of eating disorders would help to reconfigure the existing notions of eating disorders as a mere cultural problem that happens to women who are obsessed with body perfection and fashion.

Overview of the Book

Each chapter of this book offers a reading of eating disorders in women anchored on historical, literary, medical, biocultural, or feminist viewpoints. By the end, the aim of the book is to have formed a multi-perspectival understanding of the origin and spread of eating disorders and its impact on women. Chapter 1 initiates the discussion of comics and eating disorders by offering an attempt to justify the suitability of graphic medicine as one of the best modes to discuss eating disorder experiences. Besides tracking the history of graphic medicine, this chapter also provides a brief review of the historical engagement of comics medium with healthcare practices.

Chapter 2 presents the biocultural model as one of the most appropriate models to understand eating disorders with multidetermined etiology, and affirms the relevance of the biocultural model as the central theoretical scaffold of this book. It gives a detailed introduction to the clinical and cultural evolution of eating disorders beginning from the fourteenth century. This chapter also aims to review various explanatory models of eating disorders, the lacunae in each of them, and the suitability of the biocultural model of illness.

Chapter 3, in addition to investigating how eating disorders, especially anorexia, develop in young females as a consequence of cultural dogmas disseminated by family, peer groups, society, and media, also offers an analysis of the unique strengths of comics medium in portraying corporeal complications. Using the theoretical postulates of Beauvoir and Bordo, and through a close reading of *Lighter Than My Shadow* and *Tyranny*, this chapter delineates eating disorders as a bodily manifestation of a cultural problem.

Chapter 4 provides a comprehensive exploration of the origin of metaphors, embodiment, the concept of externalization, and benefits of comics creation. Although most of the eating disorder narratives repeatedly use metaphors of monstrosity, battle, and lightness, the select graphic narratives reveal how verbo-visual creative metaphors can strengthen the clinical and cultural understanding of the psychological aspects of eating disorders. By drawing theoretical insights from Lakoff, Elizabeth El Refai, and Ian Williams, and by close reading the verbo-visual metaphors of eating disorders in Shivack's *Inside Out*, Fairfield's *Tyranny*, and Green's *Lighter*, this chapter investigates how creative metaphors help female graphic pathographers in representing various underexplored dimensions of their eating disorder experiences.

Chapter 5, by close reading *Lighter Than My Shadow, Lucille, Inside Out, Tyranny,* and *The House That Groaned*, examines the largely underexplored correlation between abjection and the etiology of eating disorders in women. While the existing literature on eating disorders has given repeated attention only to certain cultural or clinical aspects, these graphic narratives draw the reader's attention to how abjection instigated by bodily transformations during puberty or a deeply feminine experience of menstruation could lead to eating disorders. In addition, this chapter also explores various ways in which comics medium enable an effective articulation of the sufferers' corporeal and psychological agonies.

Last, the book concludes by emphasizing the significance of biocultures and graphic medicine in attaining a holistic understanding of women's eating disorder experiences. In its totality, the book argues that humanistic understanding of eating disorders based on socio-cultural factors is as important as its biomedical understanding. Hence, the major goal of this book is to promulgate that graphic medicine helps to bring forth unique yet truthful representations of the marginalized and vulnerable selves of women with eating disorders and forge novel understandings of its causes using comics.

Works Cited

Davies, Caroline. "Doctors' Failings on Eating Disorders 'Are Costing Lives'." *The Guardian*, 18 June 2019, www.theguardian.com/society/2019/jun/18/doctors-failings-on-eating-disorders-are-costing-lives. Accessed 28 June 2019.

Foye, Una et al. "'The Body is a Battleground for Unwanted and Unexpressed Emotions': Exploring Eating Disorders and the Role of Emotional Intelligence." *Eating Disorders*, vol. 27, no. 3, 2019, pp. 321–342.

Lewis, Amy. "Researchers Explore the Genetics of Eating Disorders." *The Scientist Magazine*, 1 Jan. 2019, www.the-scientist.com/notebook/researchers-explorethe-genetics-of-eating-disorders-65237. Accessed 26 June 2019.

Meskin, Aron and Roy T Cook (eds.), *The Art of Comics: A Philosophical Approach*. Blackwell Publishing, pp. 68–84.

Sousanis, Nick. "Comics–Expanding Narrative Possibilities, Integrating into the Classroom." *Spin Weave and Cut*, 2015, http://spinweaveandcut.com/wp-content/uploads/2015/03/Sousanis-SPI-presentation-w-PICS.pdf. Accessed 9 July 2019.

Wegner, Gesine. "Reflections on the Boom of Graphic Pathography: The Effects and Affects of Narrating Disability and Illness in Comics." *Journal of Literary & Cultural Disability Studies,* vol. 14, no. 1, 2019, pp. 57–74.

1 A Prologue to Graphic Medicine

Graphic medicine is an approach that advocates the creative expression of critical health conditions through comics medium. As an offshoot of several altruistic movements, such as narrative medicine, medical humanities, and health humanities, graphic medicine was formulated as a means to express the voice of marginalized sufferers within and beyond medical fraternity. While giving equal respect to the subjective experiences of patients, physicians, and caregivers, graphic medicine provides numerous ways of representing affective truths about their illness conditions. Thus, by yoking together medicine and comics, graphic medicine fosters an empathetic attitude towards human conditions. The present chapter traces the evolution of graphic medicine from the historical nexus of comics and medicine, through narrative medicine, to health humanities, and introduces graphic medicine and rationalizes some of its unique aspects and cultural roles.

Medical Humanities: Towards the Humanization of Medical Science

It was in 1948 that the term medical humanities appeared first when George Sarton, founder and editor of the journal *ISIS*, used it in his response to an article titled "A History of Scientific English" by Edmund Andrews. Sarton's use of the term medical humanities was more inclined to the history of science, identified as an "an endeavor that centered on the task of understanding science and medicine in all cultures and all periods through a disciplined study of its working methods, assumptions, language, literature and philosophy" (Hurwitz 672). Sarton believed in the essentiality of the humanization of science and later on various medical universities such as Cambridge University started conducting literature courses. Against the reductionist scientific understanding of an ill person offered by medical science, literature courses provided medical students with "whole person understanding" (Downie 93) and helped them in grasping the reality that doctors like all other human beings are fallible by nature (Barber 78). While in the UK, physicians like Anthony Moore, Robin Downie, and Hugh Barber helped in the development of the nexus of medicine and humanities, Robert Coles promoted the value of literary reading among medical trainees in the USA.

In 1967, Penn State University in Hershey became the first medical school in the USA to have a Humanities Department and offer medical humanities courses. Their curriculum "focused on engendering better understanding of families, their resources within communities, the influence of lifestyle and behavior on the prevalence and impact of disease, and on philosophical, spiritual and ethical aspects of healthcare" (Hurwitz 673). In the UK, the Centre for Philosophy and Health Care at the University of Swansea was the first medical unit in 1997 to offer a postgraduate degree in Medical Humanities anchored on "history, medical anthropology and sociology, literature, visual arts, politics, social policy and theology" (Hurwitz 673). While medical humanities was initially formulated to help medical students in attaining a better understanding of various issues related to ethics, it was Rita Charon's narrative medicine movement that took medical humanities to a higher plane. Charon expanded the frontiers of medial humanities by offering a space for patients, which was an attempt towards fulfilling the higher task of the 'humanization of science' which Sarton envisioned during the inception of medical humanities in the 1940s.

Narrative Medicine: Understanding the Ordeals of Illness

Pioneered by Rita Charon, narrative medicine emerged in the 1970s as a method of "clinical practice fortified by narrative competence—the capacity to recognize, absorb, metabolize, interpret, and be moved by stories of illness" (Charon 1265). Offering "healthcare professionals with practical wisdom in comprehending what patients endure in illness and what they themselves undergo in the care of the sick" (Charon vii), narrative medicine foregrounded for the first time that without a practice of listening to the sufferer's subjective experiences medical science is just insufficient in facilitating a holistic experience of recovery to patients. As Charon rightly observes, "a scientifically competent medicine alone cannot help a patient grapple with the loss of health and find meaning in illness and dying" (1). Charon's approach taught healthcare professionals to listen "expertly and attentively to extraordinarily complicated narratives" of patients or caregivers, expressed through "words, gestures, silences, tracings, images, laboratory test results, and changes in the body" (4).

Predictably, together with seminal works published during this decade on illness and suffering, narrative medicine not only exposed the limitations and the vested authority of expert knowledge but also expanded a new way of understanding patient's subjectivity. Thus, urging to foster a culture of listening, narrative medicine goaded medical community "to understand as best they can the ordeals of illness, to honor the meanings of their patients' narratives of illness, and to be moved by what they behold so that they can act on their patients' behalf" (Charon 3). While bringing patients' experiences to the vanguard of medical science, narrative medicine also offered myriad ways of understanding illness as a disruptive experience rather than as a clinical entity, thereby successfully tethering the ideologically differing poles of experience and empiricism.

Spectacles of Suffering: Representation of Illness across Media

Some of the popular representations of illnesses and pain across various artistic media are Frida Kahlo's painting *The Wounded Deer*, which is about her harrowing medical experiences. Similarly, Michelangelo's *La Pieta* is a nonpareil illustration of ineffable trauma sculpted in marble. Likewise, most of John Keats's poems with melancholic lure are achingly beautiful expressions of his TB experience. In music, Demi Lovato's songs also share similar thematic moorings of illness. Marvelyn Brown's HIV experience chronicled as *The Naked Truth* (2008) reinforces the theme of illness representation in textual narratives. When considering movies as yet another medium of powerful expression of illness experience, Ron Howard's *A Beautiful Mind* (2001) is an intense depiction of schizophrenia that cannot be overlooked. Among performative art forms, there are dance choreographies with illness themes by maestros like Bill T. John. In photography, NGOs such as Keith Berr's 'Flashes of Hope,' which utilizes creative photography for sharing cancer experiences, attempt to alter the way children with terminal illnesses see themselves.

While the above mentioned artworks are examples of the representation of illness and pain across verbal or visual media, there are comics on illness experiences, using both verbal and visual media. Unlike other artistic media, comics has unbridled communicative potentials and lack of temporal constraints or spatial restraints. As Amy Chandler observes "[i]llness narratives have traditionally been used as a conceptual tool for exploring experiences of chronic illness or disease", however, comics' engagement with illness is idiosyncratic and extra forceful as it creatively deploys the medium-specific strengths of both visual and verbal media of expression (111). In essence, the structural features of comics make it easy for sub-genres like graphic medicine to depict disruptive and degenerative human conditions in a concise yet effective way. Interestingly, long before the dawn of modern age comics, it was used by medical professionals in the first half of the twentieth century.

Comics Medium and Healthcare

In his article titled "Medical History for the Masses: How American Comic Books Celebrated Heroes of Medicine in the 1940s," Bert Hansen observes that comics was used in the early 1900s to "popularize scientific and medical ideas, to celebrate the achievements of medical research, to encourage medical science as a career choice, and to show medicine as a humane and noble enterprise" (148). Tracing the popularity of medical comics in the 1930s and 1940s, Hansen highlights that comics was then an influential medium, mature enough to communicate the achievements of medical science and powerful enough to develop a passion for medical careers in young minds. Under the instrumental influence of medical historians like Paul de Kruif and Harvey Cushing, medical comics about famous scientists and healthcare practitioners developed into a popular genre called "true adventures" (Hansen 148) with the publication of *True Comics* in April 1941. While mainstream comics idolized fictional superheroes such as Superman and Batman, *True Comics* celebrated the inspiring lives of personalities such as Louis Pasteur, Walter Reed, and many wonder women in history, among others. Although the genre "declined and disappeared" (Hansen 161) after the 1950s, the popularity of *True Comics* was instrumental in comics—which had been initially denigrated as a juvenile medium—gaining respect as a potent medium. While comics medium has been used by medical professionals as early as 1900s, it was only in the 1970s that women started using comics as a mode of self-expression.

Comics, Women, and the Counterculture

It was in the latter half of the 1960s and early 1970s that women artists started publishing autobiographical comics on taboo topics such as sex, female sexuality, gender equality, abortion, sexual/reproductive rights, beauty, and body image with the advent of the second wave of countercultural comics. The success of *It Ain't Me Babe* (1970), the first underground comic by Trina Robbins' and Willy Mendes, led to the publication of the first female underground comic series, *Wimmin's Comix* (1972–1992). According to Køhlert, *Wimmin's Comix* "opened a cultural space for women to draw and publish comics" (25). It focused on politics, homosexuality, and other feminist concerns and inspired many female comic artists to do autobiographical graphic narratives. Similarly, *Tits 'n' Clits Comix* (1972) and *Abortion Eve* (1973) by Joyce Farmer and Lyn Chevli dealt with certain serious female concerns including menstruation, unwanted pregnancy, contraceptives, and sex education. Although underground comix lost popularity by 1980s, it is interesting to see that the female comic artists were preparing the grounds for future depictions and autobiographical graphiations of themes related to femininity, sexuality, body, beauty, health, and illness conditions. For instance, Aline Kominsky Crumb's "Goldie: A Neurotic Woman" (1972) is a perfect depiction of female body image crisis which is a central aspect of eating disorders in women.

Following the female underground comic artists, today there is a multitude of women artists including notable figures like Alison Bechdel, Lynda Barry, Marjane Satrapi, Sophie Crumb, Ellen Forney making significant contributions to the field of comics. Deviating from the self-expressive and pedagogical motives of the underground comix culture, comics medium is widely used today as a mode of life writing to depict harrowing experiences related to illness, body, and trauma. According to Hilary Chute, "the stories to which women's graphic narrative is today dedicated are often traumatic" because "the cross-discursive form of comics is apt for expressing that difficult register, which is central to its importance as an innovative genre of life writing"(2). In Susie Bright's observation, "there's literally no other place beside comix where you can find women speaking the truth and using their pictures to show you, in vivid detail, what it means to live your life outside of the stereotypes and delusions" (7). Essentially, the female comic artists of the underground comix era taught the female graphic artists and pathographers to use comics as an efficient mode of expressing/externalizing experiential realities.

Thus, the cultural association between comics and healthcare was already established before the rise of graphic medicine. Relying heavily on the adeptness of comics as a significant "resource for communicating a range of issues broadly termed 'medical', " graphic medicine facilitates "complex and powerful analysis of illness, medicine, and disability and a rethinking of the boundaries of 'health'" (Czerwiec n.p). With the synergetic interflow of both verbal and visual components in comics, graphic medicine creatively embraces the lived experiences of sufferers and idiosyncratically manifests their subjective experiences.

Graphic Medicine: Definition and Scope

Graphic medicine, which has been identified as a productive tool, emerged from the phenomenal coalescing of the medium of comics and the practices of healthcare that bridge the known and unknown realms of illness conditions. It utilizes the creative droit and the affordances of the comics medium, allowing an exploration of multiple meanings of illness and disease. With the primary objective of sharing and legitimizing affective truths constituted in illness and suffering, graphic medicine emphasizes the phenomenological and intimate aspects of such experiences and emotions. It foregrounds unique experiential truths that are hitherto unacknowledged through the concurrent portrayal of the vulnerability of the doctor, the helplessness of the patient, and the challenges of the caregiver. In the seminal indenture *Graphic Medicine Manifesto*, Williams observes this correlation of graphic medicine with the aims of narrative medicine thus: "graphic medicine combines the principles of narrative medicine with an exploration of the visual systems of comic art, interrogating the representation of physical and emotional signs and symptoms within the medium" (1). As Squier contends "while narrative medicine focuses on the textual and verbal, graphic medicine can access those aspects of illness and medicine that we experience visually and spatially, as enduring, if intractable, aspects of the patient's experience" (Czerwiec 46). Put differently, exploiting the medium-specific uniqueness of comics such as panels, gutters, iconic images, speech, and thought balloons, graphic medicine narrates as well as *visibilizes* the experiential realities of illness conditions.

As an "interdisciplinary field which explores comics' distinctive engagement with and performance of illness experience"

(Venkatesan 94), graphic medicine not only illuminates the lacunae in medical knowledge but also fills the interstices with the veristic portrayal of experiences. Graphic pathographies are becoming alternate founts of knowledge on subjective experiences of illness as graphic pathographies contain "precisely the information that is left out of or never considered for inclusion in textbooks" (Czerwiec 132). Also, graphic medicine is used in disability studies, women's studies, science and technology studies, and environmental studies, among others (Czerwiec 49–52). Thus, by offering numerous explications of biomedical approaches as well as its lack of consociation with the experience of the sufferer, graphic medicine validates itself as an alternate source of knowledge.

Conclusion

Graphic medicine emerges at the crossroads of health humanities and narrative medicine, and negotiates various illness experiences by transcending the boundaries of biomedicine and the cultural nuances of illness and health. Through its intrinsic yet authentic portrayal of subjective experiential truths from multiple perspectives, graphic medicine demonstrates how patients, caregivers, and not just healthcare professionals can contribute substantially to the holistic understanding of medical conditions. Essentially, by utilizing the structural affordances of the medium of comics, graphic medicine creates an intricate relationship between doctors, patients, and caregivers and thus produces an alternative knowledge system. When used as a pedagogical tool, graphic medicine narratives enable effectual communication of information and also enhance the clinical and communicative capabilities of future physicians when practiced in medical school. In a similar vein, comics creation also aids medical students in expressing their medical school experience with a creative scintilla. Also, by creating narrative spaces to be self-reflective, graphic medicine enables authors to access their inner realms that are fragmented by traumatic experiences, thereby effectuating its therapeutic goals. Similarly, by allowing subjugated voices to be heard and suppressed perspectives to be shared, graphic medicine forms an emotional community by bringing together individuals of similar experiences, thereby extending empathy and support. While narrative medicine is limited in many ways to the verbal media, graphic medicine facilitates access to unutterable experiences of illnesses through verbal and visual methods.

Further, as comics is a "powerful medium to bring the biocultural analyses of medicine, as well as health humanities, to a wide audience," it could be utilized to create innovative ways to perceive the existing knowledge on certain disorder conditions such as eating disorders (Czerwiec 46). Grounded on the multi-modal narrative possibilities of the comics medium, graphic medicine effectively engages issues concerning embodiment and externalization of bodily trauma. While art theorists like Rosalind Krauss lament that "contemporary art has entered the 'post-medium condition,'" comics is an exceptional form that is "deeply rooted in the specificity of its medium as a source of cultural, aesthetic, and political significance" (Chute 5). Accordingly, the select graphic medicine narratives in this book demonstrate various underexplored themes related to the feminal experience of eating disorders and provide a deeper understanding of the biocultural dimension of eating disorders. In essence, this book is an exploration of how graphic medicine, as a significant mode of artistic expression facilitates a circumstantial understanding of the female body/mind caught in a complex farrago of culture, gender, and eating disorders.

Works Cited

Barber, Hugh. *The Rewards of Medicine and Other Essays*. HK Lewis, 1959.

Bright, Susie. "Introduction." *Twisted Sisters 2: Drawing the Line*, edited Noomin D, Kitchen Sink, 1995, p. 7.

Chandler, Amy. "Narrating the Self-Injured Body." *Medical Humanities*, vol. 40, 2014, pp. 111–116.

Charon, Rita. *Narrative Medicine: Honoring the Stories of Illness*. The Oxford UP, 2006.

Chute, Hilary. *Graphic Women: Life Narrative and Contemporary Comics*. Columbia UP, 2010.

Czerwiec, MK et al. *Graphic Medicine Manifesto*. The Pennsylvania State UP, 2015.

Downie Robin. "Literature and Medicine." *Journal of Medical Ethics: Medical Humanities*, vol. 17, 1991, pp. 93–98.

Hansen, Bert. "Medical History for the Masses: How American Comic Books Celebrated Heroes of Medicine in the 1940s." *Bulletin of the History of Medicine*, vol. 78, no. 1, 2004, pp. 148–191.

Hurwitz, Brian. "Medical Humanities: Lineage, Excursionary Sketch and Rationale." *Journal of Medical Ethics*, vol. 39, no. 11, 2013, pp. 672–674.

Køhlert, Byrn Frederik. *Serial Selves: Identity and Representation in Autobiographical Comics*. Rutgers UP, 2019.

Sarton George, Frances Siegel. "Seventy-First Critical Bibliography of the History and Philosophy of Science and of the History of Civilization (to October I 947)." *ISIS*, vol. 39, no. ½, 1948, pp. 70–139.

Venkatesan, Sathyaraj. "Graphic Medicine Manifesto, by MK Czerwiec, Ian Williams, Susan Merrill Squier, Michael J. Green, Kimberly R. Myers, and Scott T. Smith." *Journal of Graphic Novels and Comics*, vol. 7, no. 1, 2016, pp. 93–94.

2 Clinical Evolution of Eating Disorders and the Rise of the Biocultures

Followed by the biomedical identification of anorexia in the nineteenth century, various explanatory models emerged trying to rationalize the etiology of eating disorders using prominent theoretical notions related to psychiatry, culture, and feminism, to name a few. But each model was an attempt to limit the etiology of eating disorders to any one of the popular models without considering the possibility of cumulative impact of various factors. Unsurprisingly, due to the lack of attention to the multidimensional etiology of eating disorders, none of these models could adequately explain "the current rash of eating disorders in the long history of female food refusal" (Brumberg 26). Eluding the collective role of culture and biology in the development of eating disorders in women, biomedicine continues to see eating disorders as psychiatric problems for which cultural factors are mere triggers. However, any discussion on eating disorders in women necessitates the analysis of culture since eating disorders are primarily seen in women, and that female identity is essentially a cultural construct. Therefore, expounding some of the major limitations of the prevalent theoretical models, this chapter argues that a theoretical model like the biocultures that gives equal prominence to cultural factors along with medical causes is necessary to make a holistic perception of eating disorders in women. Drawing theoretical insights from Joan Jacob Brumberg, Lennard J. Davis, and David B. Morris, this chapter also analyses how graphic medicine adds significant knowledge about the cultural causes of eating disorders aspects such as influence of family, media, and peer pressure, among others. Further, this chapter also (a) presents a brief overview of the cultural and clinical history of eating disorders, (b) introduces the three major medical classifications of eating disorders, and (c) traces the historical overlying of science and culture. In essence, this chapter not only aims to present the biocultural approach as a fitting theoretical model to explain the multifactorial origin of eating disorders but also lays bare the reason for choosing it as the theoretical foundation for this book on women, eating disorders, and graphic medicine.

Chronicles of Starvation: A Cultural History of Eating Disorders

To emphasize the socio-cultural situatedness of self-starvation, it is essential to deliberate on the cultural evolution of eating disorders. Accordingly, this section introduces the popular cultural interpretations of self-starvation that were prevalent, mostly in western societies, prior to the medical identification of anorexia nervosa in 1874. Against the dominant misconception that eating disorders are cultural fallouts of the twentieth-century women's obsession with body perfection, historical evidences (Bemporard 1997; Vemuri and Steiner 2006; Engel et al. 2007) suggest that anorexia and bulimia have existed since at least the first century. Citing Louise Rebraca *Shives*, John P. M. Court and Allan S. Kaplan observe in *The Disjointed Historical Trajectory of Anorexia Nervosa Before 1970* that anorexia in earlier decades was not documented properly. However, references to similar cases of self-starvation can be seen in "ancient Egyptian hieroglyphics, Persian manuscripts, scrolls originating in early Chinese dynasties [and] African tribal lore" (3). Intriguingly, the veritable history of anorexia nervosa begins with descriptions of religious fasting dating from the Middle Ages and extending to the Medieval period.

The Middle Ages: Fasting Saints and Miracle Maidens

The contemporary notion of anorexia nervosa is historically related to 'anorexia mirabilis' seen in female saints during the Middle Ages. Anorexia mirabilis or holy anorexia is similar in many ways to the present-day cultural ideal of spiritual asceticism. Known by various names such as anorexia mirabilis or *inedia prodigiosa* or prodigious fasting, this phenomenon referred to the practice of extreme starvation that women underwent in the name of religious piety. Interestingly, in Western Christianity, women who relinquished food and starved themselves were considered to be closer to God, and it was respected by medieval societies as a sound method of spiritual purgation for women. In *Holy Anorexia* (1985), Rudolph Bell observed that it was to reach the zenith of spirituality that religious women of the fourteenth century and fifteenth centuries punished their bodies through extreme fasting and some of them were elevated to sainthood for their religious fervor. A controversial and popular example that Bell offers is that of St. Catherine of Siena (1347–1380), an Italian Catholic woman who is believed to be one of the earliest known sufferers of anorexia.

Bell notes that more than one third of the 261 female saints recognized by the Catholic Church who lived in Italy after the year 1200 showed clear signs of anorexia. The fasting practices of women saints closely approximate the methods involved in the self-denial of food by women diagnosed with anorexia nervosa in the late twentieth century (Bell 1985; Bynum 1991). Bell's conceptualization of holy anorexia maintains that there is a direct link between medieval women's fasting and the modern form of anorexia nervosa. He believed that such women exhibited signs of anorexia in response to the patriarchal society in which they were trapped, and that the historical background of holy anorexia should lead to a revaluation of the modern approaches to the treatment of eating disorders. The practice of anorexia mirabilis began to fade out during the sixteenth century when the Catholic Church started to see it as a spectacle of satanic influence or possession, and such women were burnt for witchery.

As Brian P. Levack notes in *The Witch-Hunt in Early Modern Europe*, "during the early modern period of European history, stretching from roughly 1450 to 1750, thousands of persons, most of them women, were tried for the crime of witchcraft. About half of these individuals were executed, usually by burning" (1). It was a time when the female body was considered as a "mysterious, unpredictable and even evil thing unless it was kept in its proper place and confined to its proper roles: chastity or incessant child bearing within marriage" (Szasz 197). Interestingly, European society believed anorexic women to be witches who "possess some sort of extraordinary or mysterious power to perform evil deeds . . . that are magical rather than religious, and harmful rather than beneficial" (Levack 4). As Julie Hepworth contends in *The Social Construction of Anorexia Nervosa*, self-starvation was intrinsically associated with "the negative spiritual state in women" and this marked a prominent change in the degradation of the religious perception of women's self-starvation from a saintly to a satanic act (15).

From Miracle to Madness and Hysteria

By the end of eighteenth century, perceptions of women's starvation were again shifting. With high regard for pure women, Victorian society gave implausible significance to women's physical appearance, and therefore denial of food or curbing any expression of liking for food was considered an avowal of feminine grace. The young girls of the Victorian era considered the ability to survive without nourishment a symbol of sanctity, and they were respected as fasting girls or miracle maidens. According to Brumberg, "the term 'fasting girl' was used by Victorians on both sides of the Atlantic to describe cases of prolonged abstinence where there was uncertainty about the etiology of the fast and ambiguity about the intention of the faster" (61). However, towards the end of the eighteenth century, fasting girls began to be denigrated as hysterics and superstitious, as it is impossible to abstain from food altogether. During those days when physicians could not diagnose eating disorders, such conditions were heedlessly considered as madness, and eventually those women were perceived as insane and were isolated from society. As Court and Kaplan remark:

> [p]erplexed by irrational behavior, and symptoms unlike those of known disease entities, ancient healers groped for some familiar context that offered an explanation, and possibly a direction to intervene. For many, their closest context appeared to lie either in the realm of madness or in that of supernatural aberrations: extreme piety, or diabolical possession as its evil opposite. (2–3)

The ideological transition in the explanation of self-starvation from witchcraft (seventeenth to eighteenth centuries) to madness (nineteenth century) was channelized by the emergence of hysteria as a feminine disorder characterized by nervousness and lack of appetite. Hysteria, originating from the Greek word *hysteria*, meaning womb, was thought to be the cause of witchcraft. Calling it an era defined by 'an ethic of nervous sensibility,' Michael Foucault (146) observes it as the last of the three eras of hysteria, where it became synonymous with nervousness and madness. In a similar vein, Elaine Showalter defines the late nineteenth century as "the golden age of hysteria" (129) when hysteria was particularly used against women. Hysteria became a metaphor for the behavior of women in many situations. According to Hepworth, "the link between women and hysteria had an established history, and had been used throughout several centuries as a means of explaining women's behavior by the religious establishment" (37). Accordingly, in 1873, disordered eating and conditions of self-starvation were medicalized as anorexia nervosa.

Deploying the existing association between feminine frailty and nervousness, "the medical and psychiatric professions employed hysteria in the explanatory frameworks" of mental and physical illness conditions, and "[s]ince anorexia nervosa was predominantly found in women, the association with hysteria became an obvious explanatory tool" (Hepworth 37). The connection between anorexia and hysteria slowly became one of the popular explanations for food refusal seen in women. Correspondingly, a symbiotic connection was established between femininity, self-starvation (which by then was medically identified as anorexia), hysteria, and madness. As Hepworth contends: "it was the discourse of femininity which bound these elements so closely together wherein the discourse of hysteria became functional in the interpretation and management of women and their social world" (37).

Though anorexia nervosa was recognized as a medical condition in the nineteenth century, it was only in 1983, when Karen Carpenter (32), "an icon of the 1970s sweet, romantic, and feminine soft rock" (Sakko 153), died of anorexia that eating disorders entered the public consciousness. Thus, cultural responses to pre-modern explanations of eating disorders differed widely, ranging from religious piety and sanctity through fear and superstition to madness.

Eating Disorders: A Medical Introduction

The first clear medical description of anorexia nervosa appeared in 1689 when Richard Morton, an English physician, described two instances of a 'wasting disease' of nervous origins in his *Phtisiologia: A Treatise on Consumption*. Although clinical cases of wasting disease were described by other physicians such as Baglivi (1700), Robert Whytt (1764), Louis-Victor Marce (1860), and Charles Laseque (1873), anorexia nervosa became the focus of intense medical attention only when Sir William Withey Gull, Queen Victoria's chief physician, published *Anorexia Hysterica* in 1873. Though anorexia was initially termed 'apepsia hysterica,' Gull renamed it as 'anorexia nervosa' to distinguish the disorder from the umbrella term 'hysteria.' A significant consequence of this discovery was that anorexia nervosa was swiftly accepted as a psychiatric phenomenon that resulted from psychopathology. The influence of this initial classification has continued to the late twentieth century and the categorization of anorexia nervosa within the *Diagnostic and Statistical Manual of Mental Disorders – IV Revised (DSM-R)*. Previously, self-starvation was associated with different traditions such as theology or folklore, but William Gull's research works moved the study of anorexia nervosa into the field of psychiatry. The 1970s marked a sizeable increase in diagnoses of anorexia and bulimia. After its acceptance as a psychiatric disorder in the 1800s, anorexia found a place in the *Diagnostic and Statistical Manual of Mental Disorder* (*DSM-1*) as the first clinically identified eating disorder.

In the contemporary medical milieu, eating disorders are classified into four subsets, namely, anorexia nervosa, bulimia nervosa, binge eating, and EDNOS (eating disorders not otherwise specified).

Anorexia Nervosa

Eating disorders are associated with the highest morbidity and mortality rates among psychiatric disorders, and anorexia nervosa is the most life-threatening of all. Anorexia nervosa ('an'—without, 'orexia'—appetite, desire) is characterized by the refusal to maintain the minimum body weight for a person's age and height, coupled with an intense fear of weight gain and a distorted body image (Vogler 1993). By evoking feelings of extreme body dissatisfaction, anorexia nervosa thrives on the victim's psychological perturbations, such as the delusion of being fat, and a continued obsession with being thinner.

Bulimia Nervosa

Bulimia nervosa, also known as bulimarexia, binge-purge syndrome, or dietary chaos syndrome, is characterized by rapid consumption of food followed by attempts to purge the body of the food via vomiting, laxatives, or excessive exercise. Although the clinical term bulimia nervosa ('bous'—ox, 'limous'—hunger) entered the English language in 1977, there are descriptions of bulimic behavior in ancient texts (Russell 1997). Accordingly, periodical purgation was encouraged as a health practice in ancient Egypt, and there are references to a condition called 'boolmot' which is a kind of ravenous hunger that should be treated with sweet foods (such as honey), as explained in the Hebrew Talmud (A.D. 400–500). The first detailed description of bulimia was given in 1976 by Marlene Boskind-White; the first formal clinical paper that remains the definitive work in the study of bulimia is Gerard Russell's 1979 article 'Bulimia Nervosa: An Ominous Variant of Anorexia Nervosa.'

Binge Eating and EDNOS

Binge eating disorder is defined as an eating spree without vomiting and is found commonly among obese patients. Yet, it was not until the early 1990s that binge eating was recognized as a condition distinct from bulimia nervosa. The reason for this has probably to do with the medical and socio-cultural reluctance to associate obesity, per se, with an eating disorder (Gordon 2000). While people with binge eating are preoccupied with their weight, they do not appear to overvalue thinness like bulimic patients. While there is no purging, there may be sporadic fasts or repetitive diets and frequent feelings of shame or self-hatred after a binge.

The EDNOS category describes disorders of eating that do not meet the criteria for any specific eating disorder. It can include a combination of the signs and symptoms of anorexia, bulimia, and/ or binge eating disorders. While these behaviors may not be clinically considered a full syndrome eating disorder, they can still be physically dangerous and emotionally draining.

Pitfalls in the Popular Explanatory Models of Eating Disorders

Most of the popular explanatory models of eating disorders have either biological, psychological, or socio-cultural orientation. Among them, the biomedical model of health and disease dominates the current medical practice. According to the biomedical model, three important causes for eating disorders are genetical, neurochemical, or neurobiological. In a similar vein, the psychological model of illness claims that eating disorders are severe psychiatric syndromes characterized by a "persistent disturbance of eating or eating-related behaviours that result in the altered consumption or absorption of food and that significantly impair physical health or psychosocial functioning" (*DSM V*). Different from these two models, the cultural model of illness defines disordered eating as a purely cultural malady. However, contrary to the common interpretation, the desire to be thinner among patients is not always the fundamental reason for disordered eating behaviors. Other contributing factors leading to the onset of an eating disorder include feeling 'out of control' in life, anxiety, depression, sexual abuse, familial and emotional problems, the need for perfectionism, pressure from media and peer groups, or genetic predisposition. While earlier research tried to connect eating disorders with psychology, recent studies attempt to explain eating disorders through neuroscience and genetics.

In the clinical explanation of eating disorders, the notion that they are pathological conditions of an individual has been the source for a wide scope of research. However, anorexia and bulimia are appearing more commonly in diverse populations of women, making the possibility of describing a common profile for these cases less likely. As each proposed model is destabilized by the actual diversity of the phenomena, increasing effort is made to create a 'multidimensional model' to explain the causes of eating disorders. However, the multidimensional model proposed by clinicians tends to leave out the crucial aspect of culture. One unifying factor that exists in cases of anorexia and bulimia is the socio-cultural construction of gender, since most anorexics are women. Nonetheless, in clinical models, the role of gender or culture is merely a contributory or facilitating factor. The prevailing understanding is that culture provokes and gives distinctive form to an already existing underlying pathological condition that is medical in origin. While many would accept that cultural pressures from advertising and from beauty/fashion industries may make women especially vulnerable to eating disorders, it is nevertheless pointed out that not all women exposed to these pressures develop anorexia or bulimia. Clinicians inconsiderately categorize symptoms into syndromes that are operationally defined and analyzed objectively and offer reductionist explanations.

Against this clinical perspective, culture is not a mere contributory factor in anorexia and it cannot be a modulator when the vast majority of cases of eating disorders are among women (Bordo 1993). Furthermore, it is argued that most cases can be situated culturally and historically in advanced industrial societies within the last hundred years, so they cannot be primarily biological or physiological in their causation, or there would be a regular occurrence of eating disorders throughout history. Additionally, two anomalies of the biomedical approach pointed out by Brumberg almost twenty years ago are yet to be resolved by medical science. He exhorts thus: "the biomedical model fails to explain why young women are affected by the particular biochemical disturbances that are implicated in anorexia nervosa" (28) and "why there are so many anorexics now, at this particular moment in time?" (29). Thus, a theoretical model that is capable of explaining the reason for eating disorders, not in selected individuals but all human beings is necessary. Intriguingly, the biocultural model can give a convincing explanation to such queries because "patterns of culture constitute the kind of environmental pressure that interacts with physiological and psychological variables" (Brumberg 42).

The Biocultural Model

It was George Engel who articulated an influential questioning of the historically dominant biomedical model for the first time by saying that the existing biomedical model is not adequate to give a rich understanding of an illness condition. Engel outlined the limitations of the biomedical model and emphasized the need for a new medical model, called the biopsychosocial model. According to Engel, the traditional biomedical approach "assumes disease to be fully accounted for by deviations from the norm of measurable biological (somatic) variables. It leaves no room within its framework for the social, psychological, and behavioral dimensions of illness" (130). Engel argued that this led to a fundamental paradox where "some people with positive laboratory findings are told that they are in need of treatment when in fact they are feeling quite well, while others feeling sick are assured that they are well" (132). He found that:

> to provide a basis for understanding the determinants of disease and arriving at rational treatments and patterns of health care, a medical model must also take into account the patient, the social context in which he lives. . . This requires a biopsychosocial model. (132)

Thus, Engel proposed to broaden the biomedical approach to include the psychosocial without compromising the advantages of the biomedical approach, so that a health professional would be able to evaluate all the factors contributing to illness rather than giving primacy to biological factors alone.

However, the biopsychosocial model faced criticism for its lack of scientific accuracy, philosophical thrust, and the heedless implication that biology and psychology are two separate fields of medicine. According to Benning:

> a growing body of recent literature is critical of [the biopsychosocial model] – charging it with lacking philosophical coherence, insensitivity to patients" subjective experience, being unfaithful to the general systems theory that Engel claimed

it be rooted in, and engendering an undisciplined eclecticism that provides no safeguards against either the dominance or the under-representation of any one of the three domains of bio, psycho, or social. (347)

It is at this juncture that the biocultural model, which considers pathology and culture, gained significance even though the objectives of both models were largely the same. The biocultural model challenges the dominant conceptualization of eating disorders as psychopathological conditions because "the psychological paradigm is incomplete, just as the biomedical model is, in that it [still] fails to provide an adequate answer to the same thorny problems of social address, changing incidence, and gender" (Brumberg 33).

Referring to the productive yoking of biology and culture, Lennard J. Davis and David B. Morris established a revolutionary and counterintuitive concept by stating that "culture and history must be rethought with an understanding of their inextricable, if highly variable, relation to biology. The general name for this phenomenon we call "biocultures"" (411). Biocultures theory, which is related to the anthropological value of holism, is an integration of both biological anthropology and social/cultural anthropology. While acknowledging that "the term biocultural can carry a range of meanings and represent a variety of methods, research areas, and levels of analysis" (Hruschka et al. 3), one working definition of biocultural anthropology is "a critical and productive dialogue between biological and cultural theories" (Hruschka et al. 4). The use of a biocultural framework can be viewed as the application of a theoretical lens to gain a productive understanding of the integration of objective medical knowledge and subjective experiences of an eating disorder. This method takes into consideration the prevalent cultural views of illness and the local practices of traditional or biomedical healing. Biocultural research involves integrating how cultures approach health and healing based on gender, class, age, education, and their own conventional experience with illness and healing. Therefore, any research on the etiology of an illness without considering the biocultural framework is inherently reductionist because biology and culture are dialectically interlaced (Levins and Lewontin 1985).

Tracing the Footprints of Culture in Science

According to Davis and Morris, the primary objective behind introducing biocultures was to edify that science and the humanities are not always "divided by a rigid firewall" (413). The need for disciplinary efforts to bridge the demurring cultures of science and humanities was an aftermath of science wars. Until the first half of the twentieth century, there was a cold war between science and the humanities. As Sarton recollects: "the most ominous conflict of our time is the difference of opinion between the so-called humanist, on the one side, and the scientists on the other" (54). Presently, according to Patricia Waugh, "we are moving into a new era of biocultural which is a complex entanglement of science and culture" (*Pathologies of the Postmodern*). One of the significant tenets of the biocultural approach as explained by Davis and Morris in the *Biocultures Manifesto* is that '[b]iology, as a science, cannot exist outside culture; culture, as a practice, cannot exist outside biology" (418). Unlike postmodernism, the biocultural does not seek to dissociate culture from biology or "to revive the so-called (or Sokal-ed) science wars" but to combine them productively to provide a mutually beneficial field of enquiry (414).

Later, cultural scientists also felt the need to "understand the process by which certain researchers became associated with calling their results 'hard' facts and others became associated with 'soft' values." They observed thus: "while we don't deny the existence of facts . . . we do question the notion that the humanities is a realm cut off from facts and restricted to the study of values and feelings" (Davis and Morris 414). A milestone in resolving the medical/cultural dichotomy is available in the "Lancet Commission Report" (2014). According to the report there were significant changes in the biomedical approach when it was pointed out by the Commission that "the perceived distinction between the objectivity of science and the subjectivity of culture is itself a social fact (a common perception)." According to Napier et al. the Commission examined "overlapping domains of culture and health: cultural competence, health inequalities, and communities of care . . . [and showed], how inseparable health is from culturally affected perceptions of wellbeing" (1607). In many ways, such innovative approaches deepened the credibility of the biocultural model. As Joseph Carroll maintains, "biocultural theory is grounded in evolutionary biology, the evolutionary social sciences, and the evolutionary humanities" (24). In medical science, the biocultural approach is relevant for many disorders such as alcoholism, addictions, diabetes, Attention-Deficit/Hyperactivity Disorder (ADHD), and Tourette syndrome, among others. According to Samantha Frost, terms such as 'transcorporeality'

(Stacy Alaimo) and 'viscous porosity' (Nancy Tuana), which indicate the traffic between body and environment, 'nature-cultures' or 'naturecultures' (Donna Haraway and Bruno La-tour), which reflect the thoroughly mixed or hybrid domains we inhabit, and 'socionatural' (Julie Guthman and Becky Mansfield), which is about the combination of forces and factors that inextricably together compose human life, are relevant examples of the productive combination of science/culture.

At this point, it is relevant to take a detour to other interdisciplinary models, such as epigenetics, because 'biocultures' is an umbrella term that holds together a plethora of fields like

> public health, medical education, medical humanities, bioethics, criminal justice, epidemiology, identity and body studies, medical anthropology, medical sociology, history of medicine, philosophy of medicine, African-American studies, queer studies, Asian-American studies, and Latino-Latina studies, and the list goes on. (Davis and Morris 413)

According to Waugh, "the epigenetic era upholds the fact that gene has a complex relationship with the surroundings and builds its own environment and is shaped by that environment" (*Pathologies of the Postmodern*). This adds another dimension to biocultures, in that the role of the environment is introduced into the biocultural spectrum. For Squire, epigenetics is "a breakthrough field that can liberate us from the idea that we are controlled by our DNA," and it is "the study of changes in organisms caused by modification of gene expression rather than alteration of the genetic code itself" (1). However, as Kristeva alerts, "it [is] not enough to simply increase our insight into the cultural dimensions of health and well-being' but there is a need for questioning 'the conventional distinction between the 'objectivity of science' and the 'subjectivity of culture'" (2). Intriguingly, Squire establishes graphic medicine as a field that is capable of interrogating the divide between science and humanities creatively and productively. Graphic medicine, according to Squire is, therefore, "an alternative model for accessing the broader social and cultural questions posed by the field of epigenetics" (128). As Lucy Serpell and Nicholas Troop observe, 'a comprehensive model of etiology is likely to include some combination of genetic and familial (Bulik et al. 2000) personality and psychological (Vitousek and Manke 1994), environmental and neurobiological elements" (149).

Graphic Medicine and the Biocultures

As mentioned in the earlier sections, the biocultural approach is pushing the medical boundaries of eating disorders by trying to grasp the fundamental cultural and semi-clinical causes for the development of eating disorders. Accordingly, graphic medicine offers numerous ways of representing subjective experiences that are often invalid in the medical understanding of eating disorders. Its profound engagement with eating disorder experiences is evident from the wide spectrum of graphic pathographies that this book has taken into consideration. When popular media fails to give a comprehensive description of the phenomenological experience of eating disorders beyond the medical framework, graphic medicine aligns with the biocultural model and touches upon socio-cultural factors, such as the coercive role of family, peer pressure, sexual abuse, and abjection, among others. Essentially, graphic medicine brings into relief the cultural norms and underlying abnormalities associated with eating disorders through the medium of comics and creates a profound understanding of the biocultural roots of eating disorders.

Conclusion

The history of feminine self-starvation also divulges a parallel history of women's stigmatization and cultural denigration. Historical records from the Middle Ages show that self-starvation was at first perceived as an effect of possession and later interpreted as an act of spiritual cleansing. Later, during the fourteenth century, women who refused food were considered witches and insane, and by the mid-nineteenth century the behavior had been urbanized and was appearing in young, middle-class women. From various socio-cultural milieus in which self-starvation in women was seen as a saintly or satanic act, female anorexics have sprauchled many eons suffering the inability of advanced medical science to determine the basic reason for a woman's disordered eating behavior. For hundreds of years, clinicians have been struggling to understand eating disorders, and unfortunately, there is not much clarity about their fundamental causes. Through various explanatory models, it was however found that eating disorders are multifactorial in origin, which signifies that individuals are at risk because of a combination of biological, psychological, and socio-cultural characteristics. While multidetermined etiology can offer a more valid picture of the causation of eating disorders, popular theoretical models such as the biomedical or psychological models limited themselves to the analysis of biological or psychological factors, respectively. Therefore, an explanatory model that can address various aspects of the disorder is essential.

Eventually, Davis and Morris developed the biocultural model, which was a cogent revamping of Engel's biopsychosocial model. Engel's proposal was theoretically informed by the general system theory, based on the idea that all systems, from the smallest discernible system in physics to the most extensive system in the cosmos, are structurally and functionally interconnected from level to level, with continuous feedback loops. While biomedicine excels in reducing disease entities into smaller units, it fails to make sense of the broader socio-cultural and environmental connections of eating disorders. As O'Connor and Esterik contend, "biomedicine breaks any disease apart, expecting to find its cause amid the pieces. That misses anorexia fourfold" because "anorexia is a biocultural hybrid that is inherently inseparable along mind/body lines" (3). By tracing the history of biology and culture and their elusive intersections in various epochs, this chapter has introduced the biocultural dimension as a productive intervention capable of addressing those queries that the biomedical model has failed to answer. To fathom how far culture and biology are interlaced, this chapter also touched on the epigenetic dimensions of illness conditions and underscored the primacy of the graphic medicine genre in offering a genuinely biocultural perspective to illness conditions. In essence, this chapter has argued that the biocultural approach is well suited to analyze the causes of eating disorders, since it has the potential to ease the holism–reductionism dichotomy.

Works Cited

American Psychiatric Association. *Feeding and Eating Disorders: DSM-5 Selections*. American Psychiatric Publishing, 2015.

Bell, Rudolf M. *Holy Anorexia*. U of Chicago P, 1985.

Bemporad, Jules R. "Cultural and Historical Aspects of Eating Disorders." *Theoretical Medicine,* vol. 18, no. 4, 1997, pp. 40–420.

Benning, Tony B. "Limitations of the Biopsychosocial Model in Psychiatry." *Advances in Medical Education and Practice,* vol. 6, 2015, pp. 347–352.

Bordo, Susan. *Unbearable Weight: Feminism, Western Culture, and the Body*. U of California P, 2004.

Brumberg, Joan Jacobs. *Fasting Girls: The History of Anorexia Nervosa*. Vintage Books, 2000.

Bulik, Cynthia M et al. "Twin Studies of Eating Disorders: A Review." *International Journal of Eating Disorders*, vol. 27, no. 1, 2000, pp. 1–20.

Bynum, Caroline W. *Holy Feast and Holy Fast: The Religious Significance of Food to Medieval Women.* U of California P, 1987.

Carroll, Joseph. "Evolutionary Social Theory: The Current State of Knowledge." *Style*, vol. 49, no. 4, 2015, pp. 512–541.

Court, John PM, and Allan S Kaplan. "The Disjointed Historical Trajectory of Anorexia Nervosa Before 1970." *Current Psychiatry Reports*, vol. 18, no. 1, 2016, pp. 1–9.

Czerwiec, MK et al. *Graphic Medicine Manifesto.* The Pennsylvania State UP, 2015.

Davis, Lennard J, and David B Morris. "Biocultures Manifesto." *New Literary History*, vol. 38, no. 3, 2007, pp. 411–418.

Engel, George L. "The Need for a New Medical Model: A Challenge for Biomedicine." *Science*, vol. 196, no. 4286, 1977, pp. 129–136.

Engel, Bridget et al. "Eating Disorders: Historical Understandings." *Mental Health, Depression, Anxiety, Wellness, Family & Relationship Issues, Sexual Disorders & ADHD Medications, Mental Help*, 2 Feb. 2007, www.mentalhelp.net/eating-disorders/historical understandings/. Accessed 18 Feb. 2019.

Foucault, Michel. *Madness and Civilization: A History of Insanity in the Age of Reason.* Routledge, 1989.

Frost, Samantha. *Biocultural Creatures: Towards a New Theory of the Human.* Duke UP, 2016.

Gordon, Richard A. *Eating Disorders: Anatomy of a Social Epidemic.* Blackwell Publishers, 2000.

Gull, William Withey. "Anorexia Nervosa: Apepsia Hysterica, Anorexia Hysterica." *Obesity Research*, vol. 5, no. 5, 1997, pp. 498–502.

Hepworth, Julie. *The Social Construction of Anorexia Nervosa.* Sage Publications, 1999.

Hruschka, Daniel J et al. "Biocultural Dialogues: Biology and Culture in Psychological Anthropology." *Ethos,* vol. 33, no. 1, 2005, pp. 1–19.

Kristeva, Julia et al. "Cultural Crossings of Care: An Appeal to the Medical Humanities." *Medical Humanities,* vol. 44, no. 1, 2018, pp. 55–58.

Levack, Brian P. *The Witch-Hunt in Early Modern Europe.* Routledge, 2006.

Levins, Richard, and Richard Lewontin. *The Dialectical Biologist.* Harvard UP, 1985.

Napier, A David et al. "Culture and Health." *Lancet*, vol. 384, no. 9954, 2014, pp. 1607–1639.

O'Connor, Richard A, and Esterik P Van. "De-medicalizing Anorexia: A New Cultural Brokering." *Anthropology Today*, vol. 24, no. 5, 2008, pp. 6–9.

Russell, Gerald FM. "The History of Bulimia Nervosa." *Handbook of Treatment for Eating Disorders*, edited Garner DM and Garfinkel PE, The Guilford Press, 1997, pp. 11–24.

Sakko, Paula. *The Anorexic Self: A Personal, Political Analysis of a Diagnostic Discourse.* SUNY Press, 2008.

Serpell, Lucy, and Nicholas Troop. "Psychological Factors." *Handbook of Eating Disorders Second Edition,* edited by Janet Treassure, Ulrike Schmidt, Eric van Furth, Wiley, 2003, pp. 151–168.

Showalter, Elaine. *The Female Malady: Women, Madness and English Culture 1830–1980.* Virago, 1987.

Squier, Susan Merrill. *Epigenetic Landscapes: Drawings as Metaphor.* Duke UP, 2017.

Szasz, Thomas. *Manufacture of Madness.* Routledge and Kegan Paul, 1971.

Vemuri, Mytilee, and Hans Steiner. "Historical and Current Conceptualizations of Eating Disorders: A Developmental Perspective." *Eating Disorders in Children and Adolescents,* edited by Tony Jaffa and Brett Mcdermotz, Cambridge Press, 2006, pp. 3–18.

Vitousek, Kelly, and Frederic Manke. "Personality Variables and Disorders in Anorexia Nervosa and Bulimia Nervosa." *Journal of Abnormal Psychology,* vol. 103, no. 1, 1994, p. 137.

Vogler, Robin Jane Marie. *The Medicalization of Eating: Social Control in an Eating Disorders Clinic.* Jai Press Inc, 1993.

Waugh, Patricia. "Episode 7-Pathologies of the Postmodern-Professor Patricia Waugh. cafeculturene." *YouTube,* uploaded by cafeculturene 29 Oct. 2016, www.youtube.com/watch?v=CWcNULx74UU. Accessed 20 Aug. 2018.

3 Warped Femininities

Understanding the Corporeal Nexus of Anorexia and Culture

The contemporary notions of an ideal female body image anchored on thinness are believed to be an aftermath of the patriarchal western societies' timeless obsession with feminine slenderness (Bordo 1993; Wolf 1991). Deplorably, the prevalent socio-cultural rigidities regarding the shape and size of a woman's body have not only generated an infiltrating sense of body dissatisfaction and poor self-esteem in women but also created an urgency to refashion themselves according to a range of set standards. Such unhealthy endeavors to gain the perfect body have instigated a series of issues ranging from eating disorders to depression in women. While analyzing how culture warps feminine ideologies, it is only natural to consider anorexia as one inevitable link in a series of consequences evolved at the confluence of culture and femininity. Interestingly, through an adept utilization of the formal strengths of the medium of comics, many graphic medical narratives on eating disorders offer insightful elucidations on the question of how the female body is not merely a biological construction but a biocultural construction, too. In this context, by drawing theoretical postulates from Susan Bordo, David Morris, and other theoreticians of varying importance, and by close reading Leslie Fairfield's *Tyranny* (2009) and Katie Green's *Lighter Than My Shadow* (2013), this chapter examines how cultural attitudes regarding body can be potential triggers of eating disorders in young females. Further, this chapter also investigates why comics is the appropriate medium to provide a nuanced representation of the corporeal complications and socio-cultural intricacies of anorexia. In essence, deliberating the cumulative impact of certain cultural factors—familial expectations and social pressure—this chapter seeks to delineate the deprecatory role of cultural ideals in engendering anorexia in women.

The Ideal Female Body as a Cultural Construct

Emphasizing the much debated relationship between body and culture, Mary Douglas asserts in her seminal work *Purity and Danger* (1966) that the body is a "symbol of society" (115). Stripped off its biological characteristics, the ideal female body is indubitably a socio-cultural construct. 'Socio-cultural construct' is a term that concerns itself with practices or beliefs that are conceptualized based on larger socio-cultural expectations or interests, of which body ideals are prominent examples. Accordingly, there is an implicit societal and cultural compulsion on individuals to "construct their bodies in ways that comply with their gender status and accepted notions of masculinity and femininity. That is, they [must] try to shape and use their bodies to conform to their culture's or racial ethnic group's expectations" (Lorber and Martin 261). For women, there is particularly an unforgiving cultural duress to follow the popular construct of femininity which theorizes that the only acceptable female body is the one which is aesthetically appealing and which adheres to the prevalent standards of body measurements. For many years, the female body has been subject to a constant flux of body ideals. The consistent shift of benchmarks in various eras has affected women to the extent that their bodies are no more their own, but the society's (Wolf 187). In their desperate effort to keep up with the ever-evolving body perceptions, women are forced to be preoccupied with ways of achieving unrealistic and unhealthy bodies.

While tracing the history of the evolution of female body ideals, it is quite evident that down the centuries there have been manifold revisions in the way every society wanted their women to be (Wambui n.p). Correspondingly, in ancient Greece and Rome, around 500 B.C., the ideal feminine body meant full-figured and plump: early representations of the Greek and Roman goddesses of love and beauty such as Aphrodite or Venus delineate that there was an obvious love for curvaceous bodies at this time. Tellingly, the nude sculpture of the Aphrodite of Cnidus is regarded as a symbolic representation of the Grecian concept of the ideal feminine body. Later in the Renaissance period (during the fifteenth to seventeenth centuries), feminine beauty was redefined according to the yardsticks of erotic allure, where wide hips and large breasts were a symbol of feminine exquisiteness. Thereafter, in the Victorian era, the notion of the perfect female body underwent a detrimental transformation from a full-figured shape to that of the hourglass figure. Accordingly, in the eighteenth and nineteenth centuries, corsets and crinoline skirts came into vogue to assist women in achieving tiny waists and broad hips.

Later, at the turn of the century, when women started gaining intellectual freedom and voting rights, the notion of curviness as the epitome of feminine beauty began to shrivel, making way for the androgynous guise. After women started becoming a part of the workforce during the period of the First World War, the first half of the twentieth century saw feminine beauty redefined in terms of straight and boyish figures. The taste of independence was reason enough for women to break away from beauty concepts which defined them merely in terms of physical splendor. For the first time, prominent symbols of feminine beauty such as curves, lengthy hair, and powdered cheeks became unfashionable and women preferred to be slender. However, in the golden era of Hollywood in the 1930s and 1940s, curves became fashionable once again. Eminent actors like Dolores Del Rio, Katherine Hepburn, and Marilyn Monroe were venerated for their tall, gorgeous figures enriched by perfect curves, slim waists, and wide shoulders. Additionally, due to the general lack of food during the Second World War and the Great Depression, there was ideally no room to worry about maintaining slender figures. True to Amber Petty's observation: "[n]obody wanted to look stick thin—it seemed too close to starving—but a voluptuous figure was also unrealistic for the time" and therefore the ideal body of a woman meant slightly full (n.p).

Recovering from the economic setbacks caused by the war, women were soon thrown into the domain of beauty once again. With the advent of body enhancers and Barbie dolls, the ideal feminine body was one with a thin waist, large torso, and curvaceous hips. In the 1960s, popularly known as the 'swinging sixties', the rise of feminist movements facilitated the emancipation of women from patriarchal tyranny. As more women began to be part of the working class, tall and slender androgynous bodies began to be appreciated once again as the ideal feminine body type for a working woman. Clothes that delimited their free movement were replaced by mini-skirts. It was in the 1980s that Jane Fonda's concept of aerobic exercise became popular and it marked the rise of the supermodel era, consisting of women with a heightened sense of body fitness. Also, there was a newly found interest in body-enhancing surgeries. Ultimately, due to the irreconcilable obsession with thinness, feminine body ideals spiraled down to the 'size zero' figure in the 1990s, giving way to super-skinny and anorexic models.

Although "women of the Romantic period may have wanted tiny waists . . . they also wanted their shoulders, arms, calves, and bosoms ample, indicating an 'amorous plenitude'" (qtd in Fallon et al. 5). When yesteryear's sculptures and paintings such as Aphrodite of Cnidus, Sleeping Venus by Artemisia Gentileschi (1630) and François Boucher's *The Bath of Venus* from 1751, among others, depict ideal feminine beauty as curviness, they also express how thinness in women was a "terrible misfortune" (Brillat-Savarin 108).

However, over a period of time, as a combinational effect of cultural doctrines propagated by various institutions such as family, society, peer groups, and media, women were proselytized to envisage beauty as the crux of feminine identity, and to consider it as an indelible symbol of their self-esteem. In that way, women were diplomatically made to believe that body is the ultimate identity and therefore it is necessary to have a slender body. Through advertisements, magazines, and other popular media representations, more parameters of womanly splendor concerning each part of the female body came into existence, and women were effortlessly made to feel insecure not only about their body but also about the way it functioned. Similarly, negative approaches towards certain biological processes such as menstruation, menopause, and ageing were encouraged and soon women started to perceive normal bodily transformations like the development of breasts and body curves especially during adolescence and menarche as unhealthy fat deposit. Before long, the urgency that women felt to reduce body weight and alter their appearance was capitalized on by multi-million-dollar beauty industries, leading to a gradual commodification of the female body. Consequently, women were forced to attempt various unnatural and unhealthy practices such as dieting, slimming, weight reduction, spot-fat reduction, fat removal surgeries, breast resizing, facelifts, and cosmetic surgeries to feel accepted in the society. As Wolf contends, "dieting is the essence of contemporary femininity" (200). Even when women themselves began to redefine bodily standards, it was the male society that predominantly hammered notions of bodily perfection into the feminine psyche.

Anorexia Nervosa: A Biocultural Approach

Critical arguments about anorexia as a cultural problem establish a meaningful break from the medical explanation of eating disorders when socio-cultural aspects of eating disorders are yet to gain prominence in the biomedical analysis of its etiology. Taking cues from Pope and Hudson (1988), Bordo, in her *Unbearable Weight*, criticizes the clinical literature of anorexia in which culture is a mere "modulating factor" which may be contributory to but not productive of eating disorders (49). When the medical understanding of anorexia is strongly rooted in the underlying pathology of the individual, Bordo critiques biomedicine's careless supposition of culture as a mere trigger factor. Furthermore, Bordo considers such an attempt to obliterate the significance of cultural forces as a "willful obfuscation in the service of their professional interests" (53). In an article, Julia Kristeva et al. also reiterate the same by stating thus: "the biomedical discourse 'blends all disabled people together without taking into consideration the specificity of their sufferings and exclusions" (57). Hence, cultural theorists tried to bring together the clinical criteria of anorexia and its sociocultural causes into a logical equation (Bordo 54–60).

Although medical science was initially hesitant to allocate considerable importance to the cultural explanation of anorexia, the concept of a culture-bound syndrome was a welcome change. According to Bemporad (401), "AN is a culture bound syndrome in which the signs and symptoms of a disorder reflect psychosocial pressures or mores of certain cultures" and this is supported by various other studies as well (Nasser et al. 2001; Simpsons 2002). Richard Gordon further developed this into a notion called

"ethnic disorder", where the symptoms of disease are direct extensions and exaggerations of normal behaviors and attitudes within the culture, often including behaviors that are usually highly valued"; that it is a highly patterned and widely imitated model for the expression of distress;. . . a template of deviance, . . . providing individuals with an acceptable means of being irrational, deviant, or crazy; and that because the disorder involves behaviors which are both culturally esteemed and signs of deviance, it elicits both veneration and disapprobation, generating a 'politics' of its own. (8)

It is at this juncture that the concept of biocultures gains import. Owing to its intricate cultural associations, it is futile to study anorexia as a mere biological condition. As Davis and Morris (411) observe, "the biological without the cultural, or the cultural without the biological is [. . .] reductionist at best and inaccurate at worst." Therefore, a mutually beneficial and insightful method like the biocultural is essential to gain a holistic understanding of anorexia in which "culture extends its shaping power over health and illness" (Morris 9). In his seminal work *Illness and Culture in the Postmodern Age*, Morris (9) contends that "culture plays a crucial role in human affairs: but its power is far from total, and biology often combines with culture to produce colorful local variations in our behavior, from courtship rituals to eating disorders."

Thus, by bringing eating disorders into the realm of postmodern illnesses, which are "defined by an awareness of the elaborate interconnections between biology and culture" (11), Morris offers a biocultural explanatory model to understand anorexia as a culture-inflicted disorder. Since anorexia deploys the "common cultural vocabulary" of slenderness and fat (Morris 12), and because it is expressive of prevalent cultural expectations from women, it fits the biocultural model completely. Resonating with Arthur Frank's argument that "the postmodern experience of illness begins when people recognize that more is involved in their experiences than the medical story can tell," graphic medical eating disorder narratives offers a holistic understanding of anorexia (6). Through drawing instances from *Lighter* and *Tyranny*, this chapter demonstrates how "cultural dimensions [are] constituent of, and 'hard' factors behind, sickness and healing" (Kristeva et al. 55).

"At That Time, Nobody Considered It": Anorexia and Familial Pressure

Narrated through Katie, Green's alter-ego, *Lighter* begins with nuanced depictions of young Katie's long-suffering relationship with food and meanders through her experiences of anorexia, sexual assault, and binge eating during adolescence. While it is challenging to consider family as a direct constituent of culture, certain cultural practices or ideologies followed by a family can be taken under the larger rubric of causative cultural factors. Accordingly, in *Lighter*, one of the reasons for Katie's anorexia is the direct impact of her family's complicated approach towards food. It is not in the goals of the authors to find fault with Katie's family: the larger aim is to decrypt certain clues that are left for readers to gain a unique perception of how family can be an invisible causative factor of anorexia. Although Katie did not experience body shaming or ill treatment from her family, the memoir presents a graphic avowal of her powerlessness and victimization in the familial environs right from childhood.

Outside the narrative realm of the book, subtle hints about Katie's unsettling experiences at home are offered in contradiction to her recurrent intra-diegetic assertions that her "childhood was perfect" (37). Specifically, the description of the memoir provided on the inner flap of the book's jacket doubles up as a peritextual assertion about certain contestable cultural practices that are followed in her family. According to Gerard Genette "the editorial peritext is an explicit and well-delimited region" or a unique space which provides unambiguous and pertinent information that may be helpful in creating additional meanings or alternative readings of the text (6). Here, Green introduces Katie as "a picky eater" who would sit at the dinner table in "silent protest, hide uneaten toast in her bedroom" and "listen to parental threats that she'd have to eat it for breakfast" (n. p.). Apparently, while these words present Katie as a kid bound to be anorectic due to her poor eating habit, they also subtly reflect at a deeper level an intense psychological pressure that she was experiencing within her home. Green's act of offering such a vital hint on Katie's anorexia on the front cover flap of the memoir can be read as an authorial attempt to draw the reader's attention to analyze the causes of anorexia from a hitherto underexplored vantage point. The socio-cultural attribute of this analysis emerges from the reading of family as an essential cultural component. Accordingly, certain punitive approaches that were taken by her parents to develop a healthy dietary routine for Katie form the crux of this inquest. Through an array of repetitive images of the family's meal times, Green invites the reader's attention not only to her picky eating patterns but also to the family's sustained incompetence in recognizing and responding empathetically to Katie's disastrous relationship with food.

Two prominent methods followed at home to make Katie eat were (1) evoking moral guilt and (2) occasionally providing leftover food for the next meal as a gentle punishment. The memoir offers a plethora of related instances where Katie depicts how food turns out to be an inescapable travail to her, particularly in the context of the aforementioned methods. Often, the arduous cultural dynamics of the family and the strategic deployment of threat and repression as corrective measures render Katie defenseless and vulnerable within the home and outside. Identified as a state of victimization, this condition "involves any form of neglect, abuse, or betrayal that leaves a child's basic needs unmet or that violates the child's body, mind, or spirit" through anything that ranges from "active abuse such as beatings, sexual violation, verbal or emotional violence" to "rigid over control" (Minirth et al. 32).

In the expository scene of the memoir, Green sets out twenty-five panels of varying size not to introduce Katie, the protagonist, but to present her aversion towards food. The very first panel epitomizes the verbo-visual dynamics of the comic medium, where Green portrays Katie's family at the dinner table while commenting thus: "we always ate dinner together" (12). The expository shot, which occupies the lion's share of the page, also functions as an eloquent depiction of Katie's family as affluent and conservative, where the father, mother, and kids are all together at the dinner table, unlike certain modern families. Katie is introduced in the succeeding panels as struggling over a plate reasonably filled with sausages and vegetables. Through insipidly recurrent images of her moment-to-moment transitions which showcase Katie's attempt to eat the dinner, Green makes the reader also experience Katie's tedium and lack of interest. As per the McCloudian definition, moment to moment transitions give a slowdown effect to a comic, allowing some kind of importance to each moment and each minute action. Here, Green successfully transfers Katie's emotions into the narrative allowing ample time for the reader to experience the same. Deploying an array of negative emotions ranging from displeasure to desperation, Green narrates the profundity of Katie's helplessness.

Katie is described through her parents' words and gestures as a conventional picky eater who takes hours to eat, wastes food, and finds excuses to escape eating. Without a lack of proper awareness about the underlying reasons for Katie's reluctance to eat food, she was overlooked as an ungrateful and impudent kid. On a superficial level, Katie is defined at best as a defiant child who always has to be chastised and steered by her parents to follow a healthy eating pattern. Meanwhile, the surge of negative emotions that she experienced in connection with food forced Katie to believe that "[w]hatever she chooses, she is destined to fail: whatever she chooses, she will disappoint somebody" (Giordano 154) and therefore she is a 'bad girl', as her mother said. This allows Katie to interlace her feelings of guilt and shame with her identity, and she metamorphoses into a kid with poor self-esteem and low body image and a teenager with anorexia.

Given below are some conversations between Katie and her parents which emphasize the invisible methods of coercion that were followed in her family.

Guilt

In the introductory scene, Green offers an instance where the mother uses a moralizing statement in an attempt to make Katie eat: "Oh! Be a good girl, Katie, eat up" (13). When Katie says that she is bored with sausages, her father attempts to convince her by mentioning that "sausages were your favorite last week" (13). However, when Katie retorts that "they were never my favorite" (13), he shuts her up and asks her to "just eat them" (p. 13). On another occasion, when Katie complains that the food is cold, her father asks "and whose fault is that?" (13), Green evinces how Katie is always considered as an offender who needs mild corrective measures. Although these words may be apparently inoffensive, they were strong triggers of low self-esteem and vulnerability for Katie.

To make Katie eat, it is found that her parents tried all possible ways such as entreating, rebuking, advising, and emotionally disturbing her. The last method that her father attempts is sharing his childhood experience of poverty, where Katie's grandmother used to give him the leftover dinner as breakfast the following day. This evokes a feeling of culpability in Katie, as she was bound to feel guilty for wasting food. Green also provides an instance which forced Katie to believe that she was also given previous day's moldy toasts for lunch. Since Katie was unusually slow in eating she was constantly jeered at for her slow pace and her nickname at school was "slow coach" (16). She recollects an instance when the senior boys teased her by saying "your mum gave you mouldy food" and "you'll die if you eat them" (16). Believing them, Katie leaves the food in the trash bin with a mixed expression of fear and sadness on her face. Thus, in a particularly complex manner, Katie confirms the fact that she too was made to eat stale and leftover food like her dad, since she does not finish dinner at a proper time.

A simultaneous reading of these incidents with yet another instance when Katie's mother tries to make her finish breakfast through a similar method of evoking guilt underscores the fact that food was a source of guilt for Katie. When Katie discards the toast saying "but I don't like toast" (18), her mother reminds her that "there are children starving in Africa" (18). Katie pushes away the plate with anger, asking her mother to send the toast to the starving kids in Africa and the mother rebukes Katie to be "grateful to have food on [her] plate" (18). The aforementioned incidents arouse a convincing sense of remorse in Katie for being ungrateful, bad, and unable to satisfy her parents' expectations of her (13). Through these episodes, Green draws readers' attention to a cultural ideology related to food and eating that has been followed in her family for generations. While it is right on the family's side to make Katie understand the value of food, it ultimately becomes a cause of terror and embarrassment for Katie.

Punishment

Furthermore, Green draws the reader's attention to a rule that was followed in their family. On failing to finish the dinner by bath time, Katie was directed to leave the food on the table, take a bath, and finish off the dinner later. Katie is seen as finishing the dinner only after what seems to be hours after taking a bath. On returning from the bath, Katie gazes at her half-finished dinner left uncovered on the dining table with indescribable disappointment and mentions: "If I didn't finish my dinner by bath time, it would still be there waiting for me afterwards" (16). Katie elucidates the act of returning to cold food that was left uncovered for a long time as one among the many disconcerting practices that strained her attitude towards eating. In essence, even though their verbal exchanges and methods appear inoffensive from her parents' perspective, an in-depth analysis of Katie's verbal and gestural responses makes it obvious that their words had a grave and long-lasting impact on Katie.

Besides being straightforward depictions of Katie's routine exercises of eating breakfast, lunch, and dinner, these instances at a fundamental level are not only expositions of the dictatorial and intimidating status of food in her life but also describe how food could become the ultimate reason for her shame and loss of self-confidence in the private and public domains alike. At various points, Katie clearly states the reason why she does not want to eat the food. For instance, she repeatedly mentions that the food is cold, or she does not like toast or sausages. Though it is a fact that her parents' have a better knowledge about what is good and bad for her, it has to be noted that the kid's aversion towards food only grows when she is made to feel vulnerable and disgraceful. Using food in a punishing way was a rampant cultural practice in the post-war period owing to the lack of food, but it forces Katie to feel helpless and embarrassed. In a recent research, Allen et al. rightly contend that "teenagers' negative perceptions toward eating may be a direct result of their parents' attitudes about eating and food" (n.p).

Thus, Green's introductory note on Katie as a picky eater who would "listen to parental threats that she'd have to eat [dinner] for breakfast" (n. p.) becomes significant. Though Katie side-lines the role of family in her transformation as an anorexic while describing her childhood, such a note directly from the author adds complexity to the reader's understanding of anorexia as a disorder emerging from culture-bound tensions. While it is reasonably comfortable to point the finger of blame towards Katie for her disruptive eating habits or stubbornness, Green subtly and cleverly reminds readers about the possibility and necessity of analyzing Katie's experience of anorexia as a battle with external cultural dynamisms to reinstate her sense of self. Resultantly, out of the constant sense of vulnerability that she was experiencing during meal times at home and school, Katie developed a yearning for a control over her food, which was an external cause of her powerlessness. Over a period of time, the unfulfilled longing for control over food transformed into an undying wish to gain control over her body and self. As Simona Giordano explains "[s]elf-control satisfies their need for power, which remains unsatisfied in the relationship with others and the surrounding environment" (154). Here, the method that Katie follows to escape "the sensation of being dominated by an external force" is creating a "self-sufficient body, which refuses everything that comes from the external environment, and which is absolutely under control" (Giordano 154). While Green shares her parents' opinions largely through dialogue and other verbal statements, she exploits the power of the various visual devices including "metaphor, exaggeration, simile, emanata, and the manipulation of physical space and time" (Czerwiec et al. 125) to communicate Katie's silence, helplessness and frustration.

Even though their verbal exchanges appear inoffensive from her parents' perspective, an in-depth analysis of Katie's verbal and gestural responses makes it obvious that their words had a grave and long-lasting impact on Katie. As Squier observes, "in their attention to human embodiment, and their combination of both words and gestures, comics can reveal unvoiced relationships, unarticulated emotions, unspoken possibilities, and even unacknowledged alternative perspectives" (130). At a fundamental level, *Lighter* not only exposes the intimidating status of food in Katie's life but also describes how food could become the source of shame both in private and public realms, thereby adding complexity to the reader's understanding of Katie's anorexia as a disorder emerging from culture-bound tensions. Thus, Green subtly reminds readers about the possibility and necessity of analyzing Katie's experience of anorexia as a battle with defying external cultural dynamisms to reinstate her sense of self.

"Neil! You Look Like a Man!": Body Shaming and Anorexia

Body image is defined as how one thinks and feels towards one's body (Cash and Smolak 2011). Interestingly, the term body image "holds the tension of a split prevalent in Western culture between experiences of body and conventions of mind" (Tolman and Debold 301). As a disorder that is closely associated with concepts of ideal body image, anorexia nervosa is an illness distinguished by extreme fear of obesity and body image distortion. Body image distortion and body shaming are interrelated concepts in such a way that body shaming is often the origin of body image distortion. Emerging from the chaotic nexus of gender and culture, anorexia in women is enhanced by body dissatisfaction, social anxiety, and shame (Stice and Shaw 2002). Body image dissatisfaction is embedded deep in the western cultural demand to be slender. Accordingly, socio-cultural causes such as body ideals, media influence, and pressure from parents or peers are identified as risk factors for the development of body dissatisfaction (Pelletier and Dion 2007). In anorexic individuals, body dissatisfaction emerges from the sense of shame evoked in response to social rejection and other events that threaten the individual's self-esteem, social status, and sense of belonging (Van Vliet 2008). Although anorexia was not prominent among children or teenagers in earlier decades, today "most eating disorders develop between the ages of 14 and 25" (Merikangas et al. 980). The increasing number of teenage girls affected by anorexia simultaneously throws light on the vast impact of body culture and beauty ideals on young adults, particularly girls.

At the threshold of adolescence their perspectives on beauty, identity and notions of social acceptability undergo a radical change. The sudden exposure to new manners of appearance and a constant pressure to look attractive and appealing, particularly to the opposite gender, makes them compare themselves with others. Simultaneously, such comparisons arouse an overpowering fretfulness about being ignored by their peers and not being successful if they fail to follow the beauty ideals that every other girl is following. Eventually, the fear of isolation transmutes into fear of body fat and causes a state of powerlessness where they feel body image correction is an existential necessity. Therefore, chiefly out of the fear of "the social ridicule that is reserved for Rubenesque women" (Giordano 154), girls conform to popular assumptions and silently strive to become thin through starvation and dieting. This concept is lucidly manifested in *Lighter,* which succinctly depicts Katie's anorexia as a malady elicited by body shaming and the subsequent fear of loss of acceptance among her peer group.

Katie's initiation into adolescence and secondary school is the point where readers see the adverse impact of cultural constructs on the female body. The culmination of her identity as a cheerful child is marked by a difference of opinion that Katie has with her best friend, Megan. Through Megan, who is presented as a microcosm of the society that formulates and perpetuates dictums about the ideal female body, Green divulges that there is a compulsion for every girl to undergo an inevitable transformation into not just a woman but a female body with social and sexual appeal. Through Megan, who is just eleven years old, Katie is introduced to the 'accepted' ways of life at the secondary school which is all about "make-up, clothes [and] boys" (41).

Defining secondary school level as a long-awaited license to explore ways of becoming more socially appealing, Megan also attempts to give a "make-over" (40) to Katie, which she refuses with a mixed expression of shame and ignorance by saying thus: "I dunno . . . make-up . . . I'm not into all that" (41). When Katie reveals that she does not have much idea about popular beauty ideals, Megan forewarns her that it is time to cross the playful frontiers of childhood to the more charming world of adolescence. Megan also problematizes Katie's reluctance to become a part of the grown-up's world by saying: "we can't keep playing kids' games for ever. Don't you want to grow up?" (41). This comes as an attack on an already confused Katie's sense of self, that she is far behind every one of her age, that she is need of a make-over.

She painfully reckons that the rest of the secondary school girls have been preparing for so long to become a part of the adult world and have progressed from the level of childhood where she is still lingering by playing "kids' games" (41). Since Katie's family, unlike Megan's, had conservative viewpoints about the freedom and independence of kids—which, according to popular culture is what defines adolescence—Katie undergoes severe psychological pressure. While others conform to the teenage norms manifested through the knee-length uniform skirt, hair-free hands and legs, stylized hair, fashionable bags, and shoes, among others, Katie is forced to follow a different style chosen by her parents which is unexciting and unacceptable. Katie refuses to go to school on the very first day at secondary school saying that she looks "stupid" (41) in the over-sized uniform. Thus, even the length of the skirt becomes a reason for Katie's low self-esteem and lack of confidence. As Abigail Bray contends,

[t]his obsessive attention to the calculation of calories, alongside what appears to be a compulsion to fetishize the measuring of body weight and dress size, indicates that weight-loss regimens,

disordered or otherwise, articulate the body through a numerical grammar involved in an eschatology of flesh. (426–427)

Katie thus believes that, unlike others, she is not qualified to be accepted into the community of teenagers on realizing that others have comfortably oriented their lifestyle towards beauty and fashion while she was just existing without knowing how to grow up. This evokes a strange apprehension that she will be secluded from her social circle on failing to acquire the accepted standards of adolescence.

There are multiple occasions where Katie is insulted for not being a girl who fits into the cultural standards of femininity. On one such occasion, Katie's friends add to the deep sense of shame and aversion towards herself by unapologetically mentioning "who'd want to rape her?" (21) if she walks alone on the street at night. In a similar yet more agonizing vein, Green illustrates the way Katie is body shamed and tripped by three senior boys at school. They ridicule Katie for her non-girly appearance by calling her 'Neil', an urban slang term meaning boy. They push her, pull her, assault, and humiliate her, saying "Neil! You look like a man!" (48). Out of the fear of becoming further isolated by friends and scorned by boys, Katie seeks her mother's permission to shave her legs which "all the other girls" are doing (76). However, her mother chastises Katie by asking her not to be "daft" because she is "far too young" (78). Katie's worst fears get confirmed later at school where the boys tease her for not having her legs waxed by saying: "Oi, Neil. Won't your dad let you borrow his lawnmower to shave your legs?" (51). All those words of humiliation affect Katie to the extent that they haunt her and ultimately transform into the most powerful visual metaphor of her trauma about objectifying her body.

The metaphor that Green deploys is a patch of dense dark scribbles containing the bantering. It hovers around her during her anorectic phase, thereby effectually vizibilizing her otherwise ineffable psychic agony. The black cloud thus graphically expresses what Katie could not articulate during her anorexia induced phase. Through the clever use of the verbal and visual strengths of the medium of comics, Green creatively depicts Katie's suffering during such moments of isolation and humiliation. Comics allows Green to express Katie's "shame and embarrassment, social encounters around food, and her growing sense of self-doubt" (Smith 207). Green's symbolic externalization evinces how comics enable individuals to revisit the past, recreate it, and process the emotions while logically assimilating the incoherent experiences into a narrative. Eventually, Katie resorts to extreme starvation and becomes anorexic as a result of intense body shaming and objectification from her peer group. Katie is forced in a way to observe the secondary school culture and assess herself in accordance with its doctrines. Read in this way, graphic medical narratives are ideal for processing and expressing traumatic experiences related to eating disorders. In her eating disorder memoir, *Ink in Water: An Illustrated Memoir* (2017), Lacy J. Davis also mentions body shaming as one of the primary reasons that triggered her anorexia. In an agonizing episode in which Lacy is rejected by her partner who admits, "I'm not sure if I am attracted to you" (60), she decides to stop eating as a self-punishment. Later, Lacy confesses, "I hated my body for how it betrayed Henry" (73). Thus, akin to Katie, Lacy also decides to abstain from eating as a result of body shaming.

"As Long as I'm Thin . . . I'll Be Invincible": Media and Thinspiration

According to Rumsey and Harcourt (26) body image combines "subjective understandings of the body including a conceptual understanding of the body as well as an emotional attitude toward one's own body" and involves "perceptions of bodily forms such as bodily size, shape, and characteristics" (Dittmar 1). Negative body image encourages disordered eating habits in women for achieving a standardized beauty ideal. More women who are "otherwise psychologically normal" are becoming increasingly obsessed with caloric restriction, dieting, and extreme exercise, which suggests "different agents at work" (Hesse-Biber 156). One such cultural agent which influences children and adolescents alike is media (magazines, billboards, and the Internet, among others). Currently, thinspiration (images that aim to inspire individuals to attain a thin body) mediated through various media is a trend among youngsters. In Deborah Lupton's observation, "[t]hinspiration is a profoundly gendered discourse" and unsurprisingly "more female than male bodies feature in digital images" (127). Thinspirational images not only formulate cultural perceptions and impracticably alluring expectations about physical appearance but also demonstrate the tremendous importance that society gives for a woman's bodily appearance. Thus, the ideology of thin is beautiful promotes body dissatisfaction and disordered eating behaviors.

Leslie Fairfield in her graphic memoir *Tyranny* touches upon a similar theme and portrays the centrality of media in creating and intensifying body dissatisfaction and eating disorders among females. *Tyranny* depicts through Anna (Fairfield's alter-ego), the negative impact of media images on young girls who are prone to anorexic habits. *Tyranny* confirms that

> the autobiographical comics genre offers artists the opportunity to represent their physical identities in ways that reflect their own innermost sense of self, often by using a range of symbolic elements and rhetorical tropes to add further layers of meaning to their self-portraits. (Refaie 51)

Unlike Katie, Anna neither had an abnormal relationship with food, nor body shamed in her socio-cultural environments. However, Fairfield brings puberty as a turning point in Anna's life when she feels alienated from her mature body. Misconstruing the unexpected changes in her body size and shape with the onset of menstruation as a condition of otherness, Anna develops an aversion to her own body. Even though her mother tries to make Anna understand that it is quite natural by saying: "you're not too big! . . . This is all a very normal part of growing up," Anna laments thus: "[b]ut it looks like fat to me, mom" (9). To console Anna, her mom gives a casual advice, "[j]ust be careful you don't gain too much more weight" (9) which Anna takes seriously and believes that her "new body" needs to be controlled in order to regain her "younger body back" (10). Predictably, Anna decides to restrict her food intake and succinctly communicates her decision using two sentences and two panels. Anna says thus: "I decided to go on a diet. I went to the bookstore and began to read" (12).

While one of the panels shows a plethora of books with telling titles like *Fat is a Formative Issue, Thin Solution, Thin Wins, Lose Weight and Live!*, the other panel shows Katie's immersion into beauty magazines such as *Ille, Svelte, Bones,* and *Thin Thin* with emaciated cover girls. The juxtaposition of these two panels strikingly portrays fat as a cultural problem and slenderness as a solution as well as an accepted form of feminine beauty. Intriguingly, the second panel suggests Anna's gradual yielding to the popular ideal of thin is beautiful. Followed by reading a fair number of magazines and books on diet and beauty, Anna is shown as having a reformed understanding of beauty. She admits that "skinny models and celebrities looked beautiful to me" (12).

Fairfield deploys a fascinating visual grammar to orchestrate one of the most transformative phases in Anna's life when she becomes insightful after voraciously reading books and magazines on diet and beauty. Using panels that are jam-packed with books, Fairfield demonstrates the wealth of knowledge about slenderizing that is available for youngsters these days. The depiction of Anna against such a backdrop of diet manuals and beauty magazines shows the artist's creative excellence in using the comicscape to convey knowledge consumption/production in all its intensity. While Fairfield uses two panels of equal size for the representation of information gathered from various sources, the third panel unrestrainedly uses half of the page to show Anna amidst "skinny models and celebrities" (12). The panel is overcrowded with scraggy women who look lifeless in spite of wearing fashionable clothes and make-up. Another distinctive aspect is the usage of stark thin line drawings in the representation of scrawny models and celebrities. Thin lines, gestures, cartoony faces, and facial features such as half-shut eyes, the absence of eye contact, among others, play an important role in depicting emaciation as a blunt reality experienced by celebrities.

Fairfield's aesthetic choice of thin lines communicates the notions of emaciation and body image distortion with precision. While depicting Anna's mounting fascination for a slim body, Fairfield strategically reveals the real condition of skinny celebrities and models using thought bubbles where they are portrayed as persistently thinking about their favorite snacks that are relinquished for the sake of an ideal body. Through a single panel, Fairfield lucratively conveys how girls like Anna fail to recognize the psychological and corporeal travails involved in maintaining unrealistic body measurements. In a way, Fairfield is stridently criticizing the role of popular magazines in perpetuating thinness as a state of perfection and happiness.

Although Anna in her media class is alerted about unrealistic cover girls and the "modern ideal" of thinness as an "[unattainable] illusion," she dismisses it as an unconvincingly lame explanation. Anna's disapproval of the instructor's words underscores the profound impact of media in shaping her perception of an ideal body. Over a period, Anna studies pro-anorexia websites, which in turn deepens her fascination for thinness. Inspired by thin ideals, images, and "an article on anorexia" (13), Anna restricts her food consumption and measures her calorie intake. Fairfield even dedicates a splash page to depict Anna's jubilation on feeling slender, and portrays her as standing on top of the world exalting thus: "As long as I'm thin, and perfect. . . I'll be invincible" (16–17). Gradually, Anna metamorphoses into an anorexic self. Thus, *Tyranny* confirms how adolescents are tricked by inspirational mass media images and messages. What is at stake here is the inability of modern-day young adults in differentiating the digitally manipulated, enhanced physiques of models showcased by the fashion industry as the ideal female body from a real female body. *Tyranny* reiterates the determinative role of media which consistently portray stereotypically thin bodies, and glorify thinness as the key to success and beauty, thereby aggravating the prevalence of eating disorders (Gilbert et al. 2005).

Green also provides a similar instance in *Lighter* where media acts as a decisive force. Followed by various experiences of body shaming at school, Katie consumes more food. However, on failing to fulfill the third criterion, which is to have a boyfriend, Katie senses that she is utterly quarantined from the society because of her appearance. Upon finding that all her friends have "started to find boyfriends" (63), Katie reminiscences with despondency thus: "I withdrew, convinced there was something wrong with me. Nobody would want to go out with me anyway" (63). Soon Katie is depicted as standing in front of a mirror and scrutinizing herself while reading an article called 'Tips to Get Your Perfect Body' from a magazine titled *Girlz*. Katie realizes that it was "so stupid" (91) of her to consume more food, which has contributed to what she understands from the magazine as "rapid weight gain" (90). In essence, Katie becomes dangerously aware of her body image and its lack of compliance with the standards of beauty followed by her friends. Consequently, Katie decides to find her own ways to be one among them, as she was "determined to look right, to fit in" (80). Later, Katie is portrayed in a situation similar to that of Anna where she "began to read obsessively about diet and nutrition" (110). While Anna consumed more information from beauty magazines, Katie restricted herself to diet manuals such as *Healthy Eating, Detox, Eat Right, Stay Slim Food, Low Fat Cooking, 100 Low Fat Recipes* to name a few.

Different from Anna who was thinspired by the skinny cover girls of beauty magazines, Katie confesses to readers that the vast amount of information about diet made her self-feeding "extremely complicated" because "every book had different rules" (111). While Fairfield communicates the deep impact of media on Anna by placing her amidst a panel overcrowded with skeletal celebrities, Green depicts the same through the picture of Katie almost crammed by food items in a provisional store while shopping. Interestingly, Katie's renewed understanding of food restriction is expressed by replacing the real name of each food item with warning statements against weight gaining such as 'Too Many calories', 'Bad for You', 'Too Much', 'Disgusting' 'Fat' among others. Portraying Katie's bewilderment and painful memories of body shaming, the metaphoric patch of dark scribbles cloud the panel. Eventually, Katie learns to count calorie, follows a rigid dietary routine, and transforms into an anorectic. Katie's attempts to take control of her eating behavior with ghastly rigor reiterate Dukes and Lorch's statement: "when purpose in life is diminished and things seem to be out of one's control, a desire at least to have personal control over one's eating (which seems to be characteristic of anorexia nervosa) may be a logical reaction" (310). Here, Green economically uses one panel to convey subjective experiences as well as objective information regarding the impact of media (negative).

Conclusion

Equally expressive of cultural fixations and personal suffering, anorexia manifests many complex societal concerns and conflicts surrounding femininity and subjectivity. Since body perfection and slenderness have become a cultural norm for women, it is generally assumed that "[w]omen like to diet. Women expect to diet. Women are accustomed to diet. Women have a tendency to get fat. Women are vain. Women are always so self-involved" (Orbach xxiii). Whether women adhere to or contest the concepts of feminine beauty in terms of thinness and fairness, they are continuously provoked by the notions of culturally constructed beauty. Indubitably, by creating a sense of vulnerability and insecurity about their skin and body, such cultural pressures to be fit and slender has directly caused a gradual rise of anorexia among women (Landwerlin 2001). The transformation of ideal feminine beauty from the "sweetly and fully fleshed" bodies of the fifteenth and sixteenth centuries to the "fat-free" beauty of the twentieth century is fundamentally a cultural pointer. Inevitably, the very fact that ninety per cent or more of anorexics are female (Wolf 181) and that women are still under the spell of beauty notions even after centuries of feminist movements lucidly demonstrates that anorexia is mostly a devastatingly feminine corporeal warfare. In this context, a biocultural view of anorexia elucidates that certain cultural factors such as familial influence, peer pressure, media influence, and body shaming are underlying reasons for the development of anorexia. As Green and Fairfield confirm in their autopathographies, the rise of anorexia is a potent corporeal attestation of the fact that the perfectionistic image of femininity centered on slimness has affected women of all age groups. Deploying the verbo-visual force of the medium of comics, *Lighter* and *Tyranny* thus offer a more inclusive understanding of anorexia. Further, parents' lack of adequate awareness about their role in the development of complex eating practices in kids/teenagers is a cultural lesson that *Lighter* offers to the readers. Various visual expressions of suffering selves through the comic medium effectively manifest the gravitas of implicit cultural compulsions. Although medical rationalizations of anorexia have changed marginally since the late nineteenth century, it remains a corporeal expression of a biocultural conflict. Nevertheless, more than the medical aspect, the baffling interlacing of culture and gender keeps anorexia complicated as well as compelling.

Acknowledgment

Some portions of this chapter are previously published as a research article in *Health: An Interdisciplinary Journal for the Social Study of Health, Illness and Medicine*. See Venkatesan, Sathyaraj, and Anu Mary Peter, Feminine Famishment: Graphic Medicine and Anorexia Nervosa, *Health: An Interdisciplinary Journal for the Social Study of Health, Illness and Medicine*, pp. 1–17. Copyright © 2018 (The Authors). DOI: 10.1177/1363459318817915.

Works Cited

Bemporad, Jules R. "Cultural and Historical Aspects of Eating Disorders." *Theoretical Medicine*, vol. 18, no. 4, 1997, pp. 401–420.

Boepple, Leah, and J Kevin Thompson. "A Content Analytic Comparison of Fitspiration and Thinspiration Websites." *International Journal of Eating Disorders*, vol. 49, no. 1, 2016, pp. 98–101.

Bordo, Susan. *Unbearable Weight: Feminism, Western Culture, and the Body*. U of California P, 1993.

Bray, Abigail. "The Anorexic Body: Reading Disorders." *Cultural Studies*. vol. 10, no. 3, 1996, pp. 413–429.

Brillat-Savarin, Jean Anthelme. *The Physiology of Taste: Or Meditations on Transcendental Gastronomy*. Doubleday, 1926.

Cash, Thomas F, and Linda Smolak. *Body Image: A Handbook of Science, Practice, and Prevention*. Guilford Press, 2011.

Czerwiec, MK et al. *Graphic Medicine Manifesto*. The Pennsylvania State UP, 2015.

Davis, Lacy J, and Jim Kettner. *Ink in Water: An Illustrated Memoir: Or, How I Kicked Anorexia's Ass and Embraced Body Positivity*. New Harbinger Publishing, 2017.

Davis, Lennard J, and David B Morris. "Biocultures Manifesto." *New Literary History*, vol. 38, no. 3, 2007, pp. 411–418.

Dittmar, Helga et al. "Understanding the Impact of Thin Media Models on Women's Body-Focused Affect: The Roles of Thin-Ideal Internalization and Weight-Related Self-Discrepancy Activation in Experimental Exposure Effects." *Journal of Social and Clinical Psychology*, vol. 28, no. 1, 2009, pp. 43–72.

Douglas, Mary. *Purity and Danger*. Routledge, 1966.

Dukes, Richard L, and Barbara Day Lorch. "The Effects of School, Family, Self Concept, and Deviant Behaviour on Adolescent Suicide Ideation." *Journal of Adolescence*, vol. 12, no. 3, 1989, pp. 239–251.

Fairfield, Lesley. *Tyranny*. Tundra Books, 2009.

Families Empowered Supporting Treatment of Eating Disorders. "Thinspiration." *Glossary- Feast*, http://glossary.feast-ed.org/7-non-clinical-slang-terms/thinspiration. Accessed 12 Aug. 2018.

Frank, Arthur W. *The Wounded Storyteller: Body, Illness, and Ethics*. The U of Chicago P, 1995.

Genette, Gerard. *Soglie*. Einaudi, 1989.

Ghaznavi, Jannath, and Laramie D Taylor. "Bones, Body Parts, and Sex Appeal: An Analysis of #thinspiration Images on Popular Social Media." *Body Image*, vol. 14, 2015, pp. 54–61.

Gilbert, Stefanie C et al. "The Media's Role in Body Image and Eating Disorders." *Featuring Females: Feminist Analyses of Media*, edited Cole E and Daniel JH, American Psychological Association, 2005, pp. 41–56.

Giordano, Simona. *Understanding Eating Disorders: Conceptual and Ethical Issues in the Treatment of Anorexia and Bulimia Nervosa*. Clarendon Press, 2007.

Gordon, Richard A. *Eating Disorders: Anatomy of a Social Epidemic*. Blackwell Publishers, 2000.

Green, Katie. *Lighter Than My Shadow*. Jonathan Cape, 2013.

Hesse-Biber, Sharlene Nagy. *The Cult of Thinness*. Oxford UP, 2006.

Kristeva, Julia, et al. "Cultural Crossings of Care: An Appeal to the Medical Humanities." *Medical Humanities*, vol. 44, no. 1, 2018, pp. 55–58.

Landwerlin, Lauren A. "The Effect of Being Weighed on the Body Image of College Freshmen." *National Undergraduate Research Clearinghouse 4*, 3 Sept. 2009, www.webclearinghouse.net/volume/4/LANDWERLIN-TheEffecto.php.2001. Accessed 18 Feb. 2018.

Lay, Carol. *The Big Skinny: How I Changed My Fattitude*. Villard Books, 2008.

Lorber, Judith, and Patricia Yancey Martin. "The Socially Constructed Body: Insights from Feminist Theory." *Illuminating Social Life: Classical and Contemporary Theory Revisited 2nd Edition*, edited Peter Kivisto, Pine Forge Press, 2011, pp. 259–282.

Lupton, Deborah. "Digital Media and Body Weight, Shape, and Size: An Introduction and Review." *Fat Studies: An Interdisciplinary Journal of Body Weight and Society*, vol. 6, no. 2, 2016, pp. 119–134.

Merikangas, Kathleen Ries et al. "Lifetime Prevalence of Mental Disorders in US Adolescents: Results from the National Comorbidity Survey Replication-Adolescent Supplement (NCS-A)." *Journal of the American Academy of Child and Adolescent* Psychiatry, vol. 49, no. 10, 2010, pp. 980–989.

Minirth, Frank et al. *Love Hunger*. Thomas Nelson, 2004.

Morris, David B. *Illness and Culture in the Postmodern Age*. U of California P, 1998.

Morris, David B. "How to Speak Postmodern: Medicine, Illness, and Cultural Change." *The Hastings Center*, vol. 30, no. 6, 2000, pp. 7–16.

Nasser, Mervat, Melanie Katzman, and Richard Gordon. *Eating Disorders and Cultures in Transition*. Routledge, 2003.

Orbach, Susie. *Hunger Strike: The Anorectic's Struggle as a Metaphor for Our Age*. Karnac Books, 2005.

Pelletier, Luc G, and Stephanie C Dion. "An Examination of General and Specific Motivational Mechanisms for the Relations Between Body Dissatisfaction and Eating Behaviours." *Journal of Social and Clinical Psychology*, vol. 26, no. 3, 2007, pp. 303–333.

Petty, Amber. "How Women's 'Perfect' Body Types Changed throughout History." *The List*, 2017, www.thelist.com/44261/womens-perfect-body-types-changed-throughout-history. Accessed 4 May 2018.

Pope Jr, Harrison G, and James I Hudson. "Is Bulimia Nervosa a Heterogeneous Disorder? Lessons from the History of Medicine." *International Journal of Eating Disorders*, vol. 7, no. 2, 1988, pp. 155–166.

Rumsey, Nichola, and Diana Harcourt. *The Oxford Handbook of the Psychology of Appearance*. Oxford UP, 2012.

Schaefer Lauren M, and J Kevin Thompson. "Self-Objectification and Disordered Eating: A Meta-analysis." *International Journal of Eating Disorders*, vol. 5, no.6, 2018, pp. 482–503.

Shivack, Nadia. *Inside Out: Portrait of an Eating Disorder*. Athenum Books for Young Readers, 2007.

Simpson, K. J. "Anorexia Nervosa and Culture." *Journal of Psychiatric and Mental Health Nursing*, vol. 9, no. 1, 2002, pp. 65–71.

Smith, Dan. "The Anorexic as Zombie Witness: Illness and Recovery in Katie Green's *Lighter Than My Shadow*." *The Walking Med: Zombies and the Medical Image*, edited Servitje L and Vint S, Penn State UP, 2016, pp. 190–214.

Squier, Susan Merrill. "Literature and Medicine, Future Tense: Making it Graphic." *Literature and Medicine*, vol. 27, no. 2, 2008, pp. 124–152.

Steele, Williams, and Cathy A Malchiodi. *Trauma-Informed Practices with Children and Adolescents*. Routledge, 2012.

Stice, Eric, and Heather E Shaw. "Role of Body Dissatisfaction in the Onset and Maintenance of Eating Pathology: A Synthesis of Research Findings." *Journal of Psychosomatic Research*, vol. 53, no. 5, 2002, pp. 985–993.

Thompson, Kevin J et al. *Exacting Beauty: Theory, Assessment, and Treatment of Body Image Disturbance*. American Psychological Association, 1999.

Tolman, Deborah L, and Elizabeth Debold. "Conflicts of Body and Image: Female Adolescents, Desire, and the No-body Body." *Feminist Perspectives on Eating Disorders,* edited Fallon P, Katzman MA and Wooley SC, Guilford Press, 1994, pp. 301–317.

Van, Vliet KJ. "Shame and Resilience in Adulthood: A Grounded Theory Study." *Journal of Counselling Psychology*, vol. 55, no. 2, 2008, pp. 233–245.

Venkatesan, Sathyaraj, and Anu Mary Peter. "'I Want to Live, I Want to Draw': The Poetics of Drawing and Graphic Medicine." *Journal of Creative Communication*, vol. 13, no. 2, 2018, pp. 104–116.

Wambui, Rachel. "The Evolution of the Ideal Female Form." *Daily Nation*, 16 July 2016, www.nation.co.ke/lifestyle/saturday/The-evolution-of-the-ideal-female-form/1216–3302262-ve24d0z/index.html. Accessed 12 Jan. 2018.

Wolf, Naomi. *The Beauty Myth*. Harper Perennial, 1991.

4 Subjective Incarnations of Anorexia

Creative Metaphors and Graphic Externalization

Disordered eating, like any other form of self-destructive behavior, is used as a method to self-soothe untenable thoughts and to share untapped and unspoken narratives of experiential realities. Although biomedicine's stated objective is to resolve the disorder, strategies to manage overwhelming emotions are rarely explored, and therefore, most of the sufferers' painful experiences or triggers are seldom reconciled or healed. To let people externalize their mental agony, and embrace the trauma of eating disorders, narrating the experience is deployed as a prominent method within and beyond clinical realms. However, verbal expressions are often insufficient to completely convey the privations of psychological troubles (Sayce 2000). In such cases, metaphors assist individuals to address debilitating affective truths and facilitate a meaningful narration of their eating disorder experiences. In this context, by exploring the metaphors that are used by female comic artists in their autobiographical graphic narratives on eating disorders, this chapter aims to analyze the power of metaphors in addressing women's lived experiences of anorexia. While most of the eating disorder autobiographies are replete with antoquated metaphors of monstrosity, battle, and lightness, a quick assessment of graphic narratives on eating disorders reveals how creative metaphors can deepen the clinical and cultural knowledge of the psychological aspects of eating disorders. Taking cues from Nadia Shivack's *Inside Out: Portrait of an Eating Disorder* (2007), Lesley Fairfield's *Tyranny* (2009), and Katie Green's *Lighter Than My Shadow* (2013), and by drawing theoretical insights from George Lakoff, Elizabeth El Refaie, and Ian Williams, this chapter investigates how creative metaphors help female graphic pathographers in concretizing their inner turmoil pertaining to eating disorders.

Comics, Metaphors, and Externalization

Narrating an experience of psychological pain through any medium is an act of confronting and externalizing an intangible reality. Defined as "an approach that encourages persons to objectify, and at times, to personify, the problems that they experience as oppressive," externalization is a key element in illness memoirs (White and Epston 38). While the process of externalizing allows the sufferer to attain a certain level of detachment from the experience, it also helps in concretizing the suffering in terms of unbiased language (Zimmerman and Dickerson 77). However, there are experiences that are too traumatic to be verbally communicated. As Elaine Scarry maintains "pain does not simply resist language but actively destroys it, bringing about an immediate reversion to a state anterior to language, to the sounds and cries a human being makes before language is learned" (4). Often, those experiences that "cannot be spoken as it is felt" demand the use of "alternative cognitive structures of the visual" such as drawing, painting, or other linguistic facilitators such as metaphors or symbols to externalize the pain (Hirsch 1211).

As per its Greek origins, metaphor is the combination of *meta* and *phore,* meaning "going beyond the part bearing," where the meaning "transfers from one [word] to the other thereby extending or introducing new meaning" (Legowski and Brownlee 20). Popularly identified as a set of ornamental language, metaphors received a radical definition and new attention in 1980s when Lakoff and Johnson revived scholarly interest in metaphor studies by elucidating the importance of metaphors as an expression of thought, leading to the rise of cognitive theories of metaphors. Defined as conceptual analogies (Lakoff 1987), metaphors would help in articulating and comprehending intricate experiences by explaining them using another familiar concept. Familiar concepts most often originate from shared "bodily and cultural experiences," and they "offer a solution to one of the key paradoxes at the heart of all life writing—namely, how experience, as something that is utterly subjective and personal, can ever be shared with others" (Refaie 151). Metaphors enable sufferers in personalizing the experience by adding subjective magnitudes to its existing meaning while universalizing it at the same time. Metaphors thus act as bridges and give "the externalized concept an image, a role about which the client can then converse. Thus, metaphor easily affords itself to the telling of the person's story" (Legowski and Brownlee 25).

It is in this context that comics gain prominence as a novel approach towards addressing and processing personal trauma. Due to the "relation of visuality to the experience" comics is regarded as one of the most creative non-verbal medium of self-expression where the "unspeakable may be better communicated emotionally and viscerally" (Hirsch 1211). Comics can help sufferers externalize their cognitive and corporeal memories of suffering/illness through symbolization using visual metaphors, verbo-visual metaphors, methodical use of imagination, and a wide range of drawing techniques. Further, the formal strengths of the medium of comics allow artists to identify and represent their inner selves in uniquely subjective ways which, according to Refaie, is known as "pictorial embodiment." As Refaie contends,

> the autobiographical comic genre offers artists the opportunity to represent their physical identities in ways that reflect their own innermost sense of self, often by using a range of symbolic elements and rhetorical tropes to add further layers of meaning to their self-portraits. (51)

This not only allows readers to have a better understanding of the issue but also empowers the patient in externalizing it without compromising the intensity of the experience. Such an activity of creating and engaging with different possible self-portraits is advantageous for graphic pathographers, especially for "women wishing to confront traditional cultural inscriptions of the female body" (Refaie 51). Since eating disorders cause severe perceptual impairment, anorexics are bound to have distorted perspectives about themselves. As a method of externalizing the agony, narrating the suffering through verbal or visual narration can help individuals in reconstructing their derailed self. Certainly, graphic pathographers "rely on a variety of graphic and textual strategies to make the illness and its effects apparent, including the narrative techniques of metaphor and exaggeration" (Donovan and Ustundag 225). Thus, comics medium offers productive ways to understand and create multiple self-portraits in the narration of subjective experiences of mental and bodily traumas. As Refaie maintains, "the graphic memoir genres unique capacity for what I have termed 'pictorial embodiment' may even provide entirely novel ways of understanding the body, both for the graphic memoirist him-or herself and for the wider reading public" (52).

Graphic Medicine and the Iconography of Illness

Although there is a proliferation of metaphors in illness narratives, the pervasive influence of 'dominant metaphors' cannot be overlooked. As Sontag muses, "it is hardly possible to take up one's residence in the kingdom of the ill unprejudiced by the lurid metaphors with which it has been landscaped" (3–4). For instance, it is a rarity to find a cancer narrative without an implicit/explicit use of war/military metaphors, stating the accepted connotation of cancer as a battle. Metaphors have a significant impact on the way we understand or respond to an illness, and certain metaphors and their rampancy have twisted the general perspective about illnesses such as cancer, tuberculosis, and HIV–AIDS. In a similar vein, while dominant metaphors might perpetuate distorted and biased explanations of eating disorders, there are creative metaphors. Creative metaphors emphasize that while the nature of the disorder remains the same, individual experiences may or may not adhere to the meaning communicated by a popular metaphor. According to Refaie:

> metaphor creativity includes the discovery of new connections between two areas of experience and the imaginative reinterpretation of conventional metaphors In order to be considered truly creative, however, the new metaphor must accord with our basic embodied experiences and be well suited to the medium and context of communication. Each medium, I argue, thus offers unique opportunities for, and constraints on, metaphor creativity. (152)

With a wider scope for using visual, verbal, or verbo-visual metaphors, comics medium can effectively register the artist's tacit dimensions of experiential truths and can help to "organize the emotional effects of an experience as well as the experience itself" (Pennebaker and Seagal 1249). Due to its wealth of medium-specific uniqueness, comics allow artists to experiment with metaphors and their deployment in the narrative so as to allow themselves and others to have a deeper analysis of certain experiences. Because these ingenious metaphorical representations are not forced upon artists, they possess "a greater degree of authenticity and could therefore be more reliable indicators of their beliefs about change" (Mathieson and Hoskins 265). Creative metaphors in graphic narratives mostly act as an artistic leeway into the intra-psychic realms of those individuals whose experiences are beyond conventional linguistic expressions. Commenting on comics' creative engagement with externalization of trauma or pain through the graphic medicine genre, Ian Williams states that graphic pathographers are creators of "new visual styles of suffering and illness," and in doing so they "might be subtly altering the discourse of health and the social mediation of illness outside of the clinic" (118). According to Williams, the three major classifications of depicting illness conditions are the manifest, the concealed, and the invisible (119). While "the manifest" is associated with conditions where "the signs of illness or scars of treatment are visibly scripted on the body," the second category includes illnesses that are "only intermittently manifest or in which the psychological suffering outweighs the physical stigmata, that is, The Concealed." The third category consists of "a group of conditions, such as mental illnesses, that are not inscribed on the skin of the patient—The Invisible—but are felt or produce psychological suffering" (19). While eating disorders cannot be categorized as purely psychological or physiological conditions, the medium of comics allows artists to use the "iconographic flexibility of the form to make visible the effects of these conditions" (Williams 119).

Unlike other media, comics reveals obscure elements of suffering in them using "various devices, including metaphor, exaggeration, simile, emanata, and the manipulation of physical space and time—all important comics techniques, some of which are unique to the medium" (Williams 125). To understand the intensity of individuals' suffering and recovery, metaphors are instrumental as they help to "follow the complex ways in which they [sufferers] had positioned themselves in relation to the discourse of change and recovery within the culture of disordered eating" (Mathieson and Hoskins 265). While the dominant metaphors of anorexia that are available in popular verbal narratives are habitually centered on monstrosity and lightness, there are graphic memoirs like *Tyranny, Lighter Than My Shadow*, and *Inside Out* that articulate subjective realities of eating disorders that are largely underexplored in mainstream literature through certain creative metaphors.

"I'm Tyranny, Your Other Self": The Metaphor of Self-Oppression

Susannah Wilson observes that

> some of the key metaphors used to describe and interpret anorexic behavior center on the ideas of paradox, epidemic,

power, visibility and polarity. And like with cancer, we often speak of anorexia in militaristic terms: we refer to a girl's 'battle' with anorexia, and celebrate her 'beating' or 'overcoming' the disease. (219)

Apart from the military metaphor, the most common metaphor of eating disorders is the monster figuration. While most of the existing representations use dragon, or ghost imageries and have loosely expressed the oppressive quality of the disorder, Fairfield is perhaps the first graphic pathographer to personify anorexia as a tyrant. She creatively appropriates an exaggerated and over-emaciated version of Anna as the tyrant whereby defining, and identifying the tyrant as the personification of her "obsession" with thinness (42).

Vividly sketched based on her thirty years' long experience of living with anorexia and bulimia, *Tyranny* is Fairfield's graphic rationalization of how anorexia can be a condition of self-imposed oppression. By personifying her obsession with thinness as a cadaverous oppressor by the name Tyranny, Fairfield offers an interesting as well as perceptive way of representing anorexia. Rather than using multiple metaphors to describe various episodes of agony related to anorexia and binge eating, Fairfield conjures up a single metaphorical expression to communicate manifold layers of the excruciatingly cyclical and overpowering eating disorder experience in a fiercely realistic manner. *Tyranny* offers a splendid exemplar for the creative use of the technique of pictorial embodiment, which according to Refaie is a "process of engaging with one's own identity through multiple self-portraits" (51).

Beginning with an abrupt introductory panel well-posited in a splash page, *Tyranny* succinctly portrays certain fatal aspects of anorexia and bulimia. Drawn in sparse, crude black lines, Tyranny is given a gendered portrayal as a skeletal, ghoulish, and ruthless female monster. Without giving any formal introduction to the characters, the first four pages provide a raw visual foreword to the memoir. The introductory panel is a scene where Tyranny grabs Anna by her neck and tries to lift her off the floor, nearly choking her to death in exasperation, and blurting out, "I **told** you not to eat, you are too **fat!!**" (1). Anna, portrayed as a bony and withered girl, wriggles in terror, with popped out eyes and mouth agape, gasping for breath, trying to take the monster's hands off her neck. By giving such a rushed jump-cut from the preliminary pages of the book into a macabre moment in Anna's life, right in the very first page, Fairfield provides the reader a quick glance into an everyday

reality of people struggling with eating disorders. While the following pages take the readers to a chronological narration of Anna's
childhood and development of anorexia after her first menstruation, they also lay the ground for explaining an eating disorder as a
struggle with one's negating self, where recovery is at times a matter
of life and death. Some of the important aspects of anorexia and
binge eating that Fairfield expounds through *Tyranny* are the initial
indiscernibility of eating disorders, their overpowering nature, providing false optimism, feeding self-doubt into the sufferer's mind,
the ability to afflict self-shame, relapses, and difficulty in recovering, among others. By providing a metaphorical identity to Anna's
conscience and inner voice through the tyrant, Fairfield captures
the conflicting and paradoxical psychological condition of an eating disorder sufferer.

Later, in the narrative, Tyranny appears for the first time as an
old friend barging on Anna during a time when she was struggling
with severe body image distortion. Anna's realization about the
surfacing of Anna's long-hidden anorexic nature is depicted as an
unexpected meeting between the two when Anna is on her way back
home after work one day. Anna is shocked to see the sceptre-like
figure, who happily introduces herself: "I am Tyranny . . . your
other self. I keep you thin" (41). The tyrant's timely reminder that
she is not a stranger to Anna when asked whether they know each
other, subtly captures the invisibility of anorexia in sufferers before
they get a proper medical diagnosis. From Anna's perspective, the
meeting was all about coming "face to face with a force deep within
[her] that was no longer hiding" (42). Thus, by portraying Tyranny
as a known-stranger to Anna, *Tyranny* eloquently expresses the intrusive nature of eating disorders.

Yet another aspect of anorexia that Tyranny objectifies through
her brief meeting with Anna is the possibility of self-shaming prevalent in sufferers. On meeting Anna, Tyranny pulls her into a conversation by saying, "I think it's time we had a talk. You're a fatty!"
This intimidates Anna, and she wishes she could lose "five more
pounds" (41). Tyranny consoles and assures Anna that she will lose
them and Anna starts believing Tyranny who was more than successful in infiltrating Anna's mind with a negative self-perception
and low body esteem. Body image satisfaction is so central in anorexia that sufferers are often bombarded with self-doubt and lack
of confidence when they fail to achieve a certain level of slenderness. Similarly with Anna, who considers herself obese even when
she was at the verge of collapsing from continued starvation. Also,

towards the end of the narrative, after Anna finally decides to re-cover herself from the tyrant's grasp and tries to find a job, Tyranny dampens Anna's spirit by saying, "[y]ou can't start work like this! You're way too fat fat fat **fat!!**" (66). The dichotomy experienced by anorexics also reiterates Toombs' observation that "in illness the body appears to be out of the control of the self, to have an oppos-ing will of its own. Rather than functioning effectively at the bid-ding of the self, the body-in-illness thwarts plans, impedes choices" (214). All of these are creative ways of explaining how anorexics are helplessly forced by their contradicting selves to use laxatives or emetics, deceive themselves by not following meal plans (95), and stay clean by not eating anything.

Fairfield gives multiple instances where Tyranny infiltrates Anna's thoughts with a negative perception about herself by mak-ing her believe that she is fat. Every time Anna tries to stabilize her-self by eating something, Tyranny pushes her back to square one. And that also depicts the recurrence of eating disorders in spite of sustained efforts of recovery. Occasionally, Anna's normal self gets anxious about her steadily declining health by wondering, "what if I starve to death?" Tyranny scoffs at her for being naïve, say-ing, "don't be silly. Dieting's not going to kill you. Don't be such a sissy!" (43). Every time when Anna binges, Tyranny grabs her by her neck, forcing Anna to vomit it all out by using emetics if necessary. Thus, Tyranny forces Anna to abstain from eating and to purge after eating. Interestingly, Tyranny thus doubles up as a metaphor of Anna's binge–purge dichotomy as well. Towards the end of the narrative, after Anna finally decides to recover herself from the grasp of Tyranny and tries to find a job, Tyranny dampens Anna's spirit by saying, "[y]ou can't start work like this! You're way too fat fat fat **fat!!**" (66). All of these are creative ways of explaining how anorexics are helplessly forced by their contradicting selves to use laxatives or emetics, cheat themselves by not following meal plans (95), and stay pure by not eating anything.

Later, with sustained effort and the help of Dr Moon, a psycholo-gist who helps Anna to "claim" her thoughts (66), Anna finally con-fronts Tyranny and refuses to be dominated by her, saying, "No! I am not going to do anything you want me to do anymore! . . . "You're not powerful anymore" (108–109). As Anna resists Tyranny's dom-ination, readers get to see Tyranny growing weaker and losing its dominance over Anna. Tyranny's falls off from her life, and tapers into a sheer line drawing that makes a way out of the last page thereby metaphorically withdrawing from Anna's life. Through the tyranny metaphor, anorexia and bulimia are concretized as psychological conditions of being overpowered by body-image perfection and obsession for thinness. The tyrant's skeletal figure, huge size, and barbarous attitude towards Anna portray anorexia as a manifestation of one's desire to be perfect by any means and how it gives contradictory compulsions to stay thin as well as healthy. Thus, using anorexia as a character in the narrative, Fairfield lays bare the intricacies of anorexia as a condition of self-oppression.

"My Ed—So Big and STRONG": Relationship Metaphors in Anorexia Narratives

In spite of its disparaging consequences, anorexia is believed to be an empowering condition by anorectics, at least in the initial period before medical treatment. Several studies affirm that anorexia is indeed a struggle for control (Bruch 1978; Malson and Ussher 1996). Therefore, with the loss of control over self-esteem women can go to extremities of food restriction to meet the unwritten standards set by society (Brumburg 2000). In such situations, anorexic habits are understood as enthused ways of staying in tune with the societal norms of normalcy. It is not new in the eating disorder literature to see anorexics refuse medication to nurture their anorexia. Often, anorexics develop strong relationships with their anorexic thoughts where they would personify the illness as a faithful and supportive companion. To explain anorexia in terms of relationships, Megan Warin uses the concept of relatedness from kinship studies. Warin observes that "[r]ather than positioning anorexia and other eating disorders within a framework of individual pathology, . . . relatedness, in all its forms, is central to people's practices and experiences of anorexia" (2). She further theorizes that relationships help anorexics in meaning creation. According to Warin:

> Negating consensual avenues of relatedness did not leave these people in a void. On the contrary, they created new meanings and experiences of being related. New forms of relatedness included concealment of anorexic practices (from family, medical staff, and friends), secrecy and competitiveness with other in-patients, friendships forged through sharing a common diagnosis, and the personification of anorexia as a friend, an abusive lover, a parent, a child, the devil in disguise, or an enemy. Some people even gave anorexia a name like Ana or Ed (the former a shortened version of anorexia and the latter an

acronym of "eating disorder"). Individually and collectively, people entered into a relationship with anorexia that in turn tempered their relation- ship with their everyday worlds. (2)

In line with this thought, graphic medical narratives such as *Inside Out* and *Tyranny* elicit metaphorical examples of patients developing a friendly relationship with their anorexia. *Inside Out* (2007) is Shivack's autobiographical visual memoir based on her lifelong struggle with an eating disorder. As a collection of rudimentary drawings and verbal snippets drawn on paper napkins, the memoir is an honest creative expression of recovering from anorexia narrated through Nad, Shivack's narrative avatar.

Like many other authors, Shivack also expresses anorexia as a monster, but only towards the second half of the narrative. In the beginning, Shivack introduces eating disorder as Ed, Nad's boyfriend. Depicting herself as leaning on Ed who is riding a pink bike, which is symbolic of her life, Nad ruminates that "my Ed—so **Big** and **STRONG**" (n.p. emphasis in original). By depicting Ed as a stylish man, the artist communicates various meanings such as the prevalent view of anorexia as a lifestyle choice or having anorexia as a fashion statement, and how anorexia is a source of companionship and support to the sufferer troubled by the society and family. Signaling the ruinous extent to which patients depend on anorexia for achieving a complacent life, Nad expresses her faith in Ed by saying, "I know he'll take care of me" (n.p.). Though Nad's thoughts have a pseudo-shade of hope, her appearance reveals her deteriorating health condition. This draws the reader's attention to the parallel layering of two realities within the same panel, which is possible only through a medium like comics. Using the verbo-visual dynamics of comics, Shivack has eloquently communicated the inherent dichotomy felt by anorexics reiterating how "planes of reality can coexist in the diegetic space of a comic—daily life, fantasy, spirit world, dream-space, myth, historical past, allegory, metaphor, metonym" (Mitchell 258). This in a way attests to the prominence of comics as one of the best media for narrating illness experiences. Even though Nad feels skeptical about the path that Ed is taking, ("but where is he going? It's getting kinda dark" (n.p.), Shivack strengthens the companion metaphor by rhetorically stating thus: "and Nad puts all **POWER** and **CONTROL** of her life into "his" hands!" (n.p.). As she mentions, Ed takes her for "the ride of her life" (n.p. emphasis in original), and eventually Ed transforms into a fire-spitting monster and dominates Nad's eating pattern and her life itself. This adequately explains and creatively expresses the dependency aspect of anorexics on their illness condition.

A similar instance is available in *Tyranny,* where Anna develops a warm friendship with Tyranny. On realizing that Tyranny could understand her unspoken worries about not being thin and happy, she seeks Tyranny's help to achieve a slender body which could make her happy and perfect. To Anna's surprise, Tyranny instantly promises her that she'll make Anna "thin, thin, thin!!," and that gives much solace to Anna (42). Fairfield gives a poignant depiction of their friendship when Tyranny caresses Anna's cheek and assures that Anna is her "very best friend" (43) by patting her shoulder in response to Anna's query, "Good! And will you love me?" (43). Similar to Shivack, Fairfield also uses a journey metaphor to explain how Anna found comfort in Tyranny's companionship as days passed. However, their friendship takes a wild turn, and Tyranny starts controlling Anna. This is evident in a brilliant depiction of Tyranny perched on top of Anna, guiding and directing her by grabbing her neck, completely overpowering Anna.

By using relationship metaphors, both artists alert readers to the fact that there is an inherent element of pain resembling a breach of trust and rejection involved in the eating disorder experience. While these metaphors may not be supportive of the medical explanations of anorexia, they surely speak volumes about the subjective trauma that is characteristic of eating disorders. Alluding to the importance of metaphors, Julian Jaynes (n.p) contends that a narrative

> generates new patterns of consciousness, which, in turn, transcend the subjective experience that is being described. As a result, the patient unwittingly creates a metaphor, the explication of which may yield insight into the patient's past and unconscious conflict.

In essence, these are two highly creative exemplifications of that aspect of anorexia which cannot be easily conveyed with such clarity and intensity in most other media.

Dark Clouds of Despair: The Metaphor of Pervasiveness

Lighter Than My Shadow is yet another example of graphic medicine's creative use of metaphors to communicate an eating disorder sufferer's psychic trauma. There is a pervasive sense of gloom and bleakness that is characteristic of the memoir, and it is expressed mainly through the greyish black background shade and the reiterative appearance of a cloud of black scribbles. Katie introduces the visual metaphor of a patch of scribbles over her head to communicate her ineffable and inconsolable psychological agony and concurrently to reinforce the omnipresent nature of anorexic habits. As explained in the previous chapter, the dense dark scribbles are a metaphoric representation of Katie's traumatic memories of body shaming and ill treatment that haunted her throughout her teenage phase of anorexia and binge eating. As Huang contends, "the menacing aftershock" of body shaming hovers over her head as a "sinister cloud of black scratches" or "dark abrasions" which not only represent "an excess of shame and bad affect" but also "materially mark the pervasive influence of anorexia" in Katie's life (300). Katie introduces the metaphor followed by various agonizing episodes of body shaming at school, where she gets teased by senior boys for her appearance that did not match the popular standards of femininity. Gradually tracing the transformation of their words as reverberating waves of voices in the initial stage and later into a thick patch of dark scribbles that hovers around Katie almost all of the time, Green makes a compelling expression of what it means to have a life-altering moment of body shaming in the life of an anorexic.

Apart from sharing the degenerative effect of body shaming, the metaphor that doubles up as Green's iconography also communicates the harrowing psychic pain of a woman suffering from eating disorders. By depicting the black cloud above Katie's head, Green successfully explains eating disorders as disorders triggered by a deadly conglomeration of traumatic experiences, memories, fears, body dissatisfaction, and negative thoughts. Such a depiction elucidates anorexia as a complex psychological condition that cannot be taken lightly. Green's memoir offers sympathetic understandings of the existential challenges that can cause the onset of anorexia in teenagers. Therefore, rather than perpetuating negative views about anorexia, *Lighter* "work[s] against misinformation and negative perceptions" (Smith 194). *Lighter* also evinces how comics facilitates the reconstruction of identity from fragmented lives by providing a sheltered space for individuals to negotiate and reflect on their past. As Williams (119) observes, "making autobiographical comics is a type of symbolic creativity that helps form identity—a way to reconstruct the world, placing fragments of testimony into a meaningful narrative and physically reconstructing the damaged body." Using the black scribbles as its most significant and prevalent visual metaphor, *Lighter* effectually *visibilizes* and concretizes Katie's frightful memories of desolation and distress caused by eating disorders.

Epitomizing the Indefinable: The Power of Comics Medium

Fairfield's experimentation with the spatio-topical aspects of the comics page is an integral aspect in the effective narration of Anna's experience of eating disorders. Though *Tyranny* may initially look like a typical graphic novel with traditional page layout and panel arrangements, a deeper scrutiny of certain pages reveals interesting ways in which the artist has creatively made use of the location of the panel, border, hyperframe, and margin, among other characteristics. According to Thierry Groensteen, the three important parameters that describe a panel are *form, area,* and *site.* While form and area are geometric categories referring to the shape and measure of the panel, site refers to a panel's "location on the page" (Groensteen 25). Fairfield's precision in placing panels reiterates Groensteen's observation that even though comics panels usually "occupy one of the places of the page that enjoys a natural privilege, like the upper left hand corner, the geometric centre or the lower right hand corner," many artists have assimilated the fact that "key moments of the story coincide with these initial, central and terminal positions" (26). The introductory panel of *Tyranny,* Tyranny's first meeting with Anna, and Tyranny's disintegration in the last page, are select examples which explain a similar logic behind placing the panel in the middle of the page so as to make the reader not just take a glance at it but realize that the described moment is significant and therefore worthy of time spent in studying it.

In the depiction of the conversations between Anna and Tyranny, the tyrant is mostly placed at the corner of the panel making her a part of the panel's framework. Often Tyranny's backbone interfuses with the panel border, giving a creative explanation of the undeniable presence of anorexia in Anna's life. While Tyranny occupies either one of the vertical borders of the panel to show its irrefutable control over Anna's life, Anna, in contrast, is mostly pushed to the other side border, often representing how she is literally and metaphorically pushed to the edge by the eating disorder. Reiterating Horton's view that "as people construct and apply metaphors to their particular circumstances, they reveal themselves at their most human, using their personal metaphoric images and resources to create for themselves meaning of the world and their relationship to it" (279). This is a unique trait that only a medium like comics can achieve so effortlessly.

Yet another interesting aspect is that it is only in panels where Tyranny is present that the border is seen as geometrically incomplete, whereas most other panels that explain Anna's day-to-day life or past mostly have clear rectangular or square shape with solid borders, and clear gutter space. The lack of finished border lines for panels that contain Tyranny underscores a range of meanings associated with eating disorders. While Tyranny has its bones or hair protruding sloppily out of the well-organized panel framework, Fairfield makes a graphic statement about the near impossibility of having absolute control over one's anorexic thoughts. Such transgressions also function as emanatas representing movements, pressure, and wrestling. As Williams contends, "meaning is enhanced and sensation intensified . . . by the use of emanata (lines or words that protrude from a person or object 'to show what's going on' or to 'reveal internal conditions')" (118). In a similar vein, Fairfield's creative use of hyperframe, which is the implied "exterior outline" to all the panels on a page (Groensteen 26), in the presence of Tyranny strengthens the previous observation. Whenever Tyranny appears before Anna, panels disrupt from their traditional framework and assume a willful and anarchic form. Lack of hyperframe in such contexts effectively shows the pervasiveness and intrusive nature of chaotic thoughts. Presenting this disarray as an aftermath of anorexic thoughts in the life of the sufferer, Fairfield allows characters to transcend the margin space as well. Essentially, *Tyranny* has an interesting internal structural dynamics which is complexly linked to the larger theme of the novel.

Equally fascinating is the manner in which the artist depicts Tyranny's downfall and exit from Anna's life. In the last few pages of the narrative, readers once again get to see Fairfield's adept utilization of panel borders in providing an enhanced perspective of recovery. Unlike previous panels in which Tyranny was an essential part of the panel structure, Tyranny is depicted in the double page as losing stability and falling off. In an effort to convey how it is not easy to recuperate from eating disorders and that they can resurface any time, the artist depicts Tyranny as trying to hold on the panel border like using it as a rope to climb back into Anna's life. However, Tyranny loses its grip and collapses into the borderless, plain canvas of the white page and tapers off as a thin line out of the last page.

It is remarkable to see that in *Tyranny*, the aforementioned possibilities of the medium are all explored using a single metaphor. Besides effectively expressing her complex psychological trauma through the metaphoric figure, Fairfield also makes creative use of the affordances of the medium to provide a deeper understanding of the intricacies of eating disorder. This in a way supports the objective of this book to say that comics, because of its formal affordances and the possibilities of exploiting verbo-visual/visual metaphor, is one of the most powerful media to communicate psychological tribulations. As *Tyranny* illustrates, visual metaphors concretize abstract experiences and "effectuate the author's expression as well as aid the reader to understand subjective realities with heightened clarity" (Venkatesan and Peter n.p.). Visual metaphors and imageries are two methods of conceptualizing illnesses, and Fairfield's deployment of the tyranny metaphor helps her in taking readers deep into the inner labyrinths of eating disorder experiences. Even though numerous verbal narratives have attempted to make readers familiar with these aspects, no other narrative thus far has provided a creative look into the obsessive other self of the anorexic sufferer through a metaphorical embodiment like Tyranny, because "comic artists are . . . able to draw on the associations of the medium with humor, fantasy, irony, and subversion" (Refaie 152).

Conclusion

Within the context of illness experiences, narrating the suffering or pain is an act of meaning making as well as therapy because narratives of experiences aid in understanding one's sense of self. Through comics, a productive intersection of verbal and visual media, graphic medicine enhances the expressivity of unspeakable subjective experiences and emotions. Building on the concept that eating disorders are traumatic events, this chapter has analyzed how visual metaphors help artists in communicating their affective truths that are often silenced within the mainstream perspective of anorexia, which is the clinical description. Bringing together trauma theory and metaphorical thinking, Berger states that "trauma theory is, in many ways, ultimately a theory of metaphor; it is a way of thinking about how some extreme event or experience that is radically non-linguistic, that seems even to negate language, is somehow carried across into language" (563–564).

To convey to a larger audience that eating disorder experiences are a chaotic spectrum of traumatic events and instances, authors often resort to metaphors irrespective of the medium. When it comes to comics, there are certain additional qualities of the medium that make visual and verbo-visual metaphors more expressive than verbal metaphors. Further, by experimenting with the structural features of the form and by using creative metaphors, artists can also express various magnitudes of their experiences that would be instrumental in forging a different understanding of eating disorders. Identifying comics creation as a form of self-restoration, Matthew J. Mulholland observes that "as a medium, comic books provide their creators a wide variety of resources to aid their mental health. They allow for expression of the self in terms of body image, verbal expression, physical action, and emotion" (43).

Appropriately, graphic medicine, which combines comics and medicine, efficiently demonstrates the communicative benefits of visual metaphors. Graphic medicine allows the artist and the reader to reflect upon experiences, to productively use unstructured time, and to enhance self-awareness. In addition to organizing the creator's fragmented experiential realities into a coherent narrative through writing, the technique of embodiment allows artists to distance themselves from and divert their own pain and trauma. The exercise of externalizing stifled emotions or memories using color, texture, drawing, and writing techniques and formal affordances of the medium clears the way for healing. Furthermore, comics is a familiar and secure medium that can be used by anyone as it provides "many safe opportunities to visually form and contain conflict" (Franklin 81). Likewise, reading autobiographical comics on illness and trauma is also beneficial, as it alerts readers to the possibilities of processing and expressing their experiential realities.

In totality, creating or reading graphic medical narratives offers patients an opportunity to confront their unresolved past, helps individuals to redefine their selves, and enhances their mental well-being. While it helps artists to express their inner pandemonium, comics also allows readers to bear witness to the author's experiences and become a part of a larger community. Interestingly, graphic medical narratives create an emotional, bio-social community of individuals dealing with similar conditions of suffering. Put differently, graphic medicine's distinctive capacity for externalizing experiences of corporeal and psychological disruptions like eating disorders creates avant-garde ways of understanding the fragmented selves and psyches of patients.

Acknowledgment

This chapter is derived in part from an article published in the *Journal of Graphic Novels and Comics* on 28 August 2019 © Taylor & Francis, available online: www.tandfonline.com/10.1080/21504857. 2019.1657158

Works Cited

Berger, James. "Trauma without Disability, Disability without Trauma: A Disciplinary Divide." *JAC*, vol. 24, no. 24, 2004, pp. 563–582.

Brumberg, Joan Jacobs. *Fasting Girls: The History of Anorexia Nervosa.* Vintage Books, 2000.

Bruch, Hilde. *The Golden Cage: The Enigma of Anorexia Nervosa.* Harvard UP, 1978.

Czerwiec, MK et al. *Graphic Medicine Manifesto.* The Pennsylvania State UP, 2015.

Davidson, Larry, and John S. Strauss. "Sense of Self in Recovery from Severe Mental Illness." *British Journal of Medical Psychology*, vol. 65, 1992, pp. 131–145.

Dias, Karen. "The Ana Sanctuary: Women's Pro-Anorexia Narratives in Cyberspace." *Journal of International Women's Studies*, vol. 4, no. 2, 2003, pp. 31–45.

Donovan, Courtney, and Ebru Ustundag. "Graphic Narratives, Trauma and Social Justice." *Studies in Social Justice*, vol. 11, no. 2, 2017, pp. 221–237.

Fairfield, Lesley. *Tyranny.* Tundra Books, 2009.

Franklin, Mathew. "Art Therapy and Self-Esteem." *Art Therapy: Journal of the American Art Therapy*, vol. 9, no. 2, 1992, pp. 78–84.

Green, Katie. *Lighter Than My Shadow.* Random House, 2013.

Groensteen, Thierry. *The System of Comics.* UP of Mississippi, 2007.

Hirsch, Marianne. "Editor's Column: Collateral Damage." *PMLA*, vol. 119, no. 5, 2004, pp. 1209–1215.

Horton, Scott L. "Conceptualizing Transition the Role of Metaphor in Describing the Experience of Change at Midlife." *Journal of Adult Development*, vol. 9, no. 4, 2002, pp. 277–290.

Huang, Michelle N. "*Lighter Than My Shadow* by Katie Green - Review." *Configurations*, vol. 22, no. 2, 2014, pp. 299–301.

Jaynes, Julian. *The Origin of Consciousness in the Breakdown of the Bicameral Mind.* Houghton Mifflin, 2003.

Lakoff, George, and Mark Johnson. *Metaphors We Live By.* U of Chicago P, 1980.

Lakoff, George. *Women, Fire, and Dangerous Things: What Categories Reveal about the Mind.* U of Chicago P, 1987.

Legowski, Teresa, and Keith Brownlee. "Working with Metaphor in Narrative Therapy." *Journal of Family Psychotherapy*, vol. 12, no. 1, 2001, pp. 19–28.

Malson, Helen, and Jane M Ussher. "Body Poly-texts: Discourses of the Anorexic Body." *Journal of Community & Applied Social Psychology*, vol. 6, 1996, pp. 267–280.

Mathieson, Lindsay C, and Marie L Hoskins. "Metaphors of Change in the Context of Eating Disorders: Bridging Understandings with Girls' Perceptions." *Canadian Journal of Counselling*, vol. 39, no. 4, 2005, pp. 260–274.

McCloud, Scott. *Understanding Comics: The Invisible Art*. William Morrow Paperbacks, 1993.

Mitchell, Adrielle A. "Distributed Identity: Networking Image Fragments in Graphic Memoirs." *Studies in Comics*, vol. 1, no. 2, 2010, pp. 257–279.

Mulholland, Matthew J. "Comics as Art Therapy." *Art Therapy: Journal of the American Art Therapy*, vol. 21, no. 1, 2004, pp. 42–43.

Pennebaker, James W. "Telling Stories: The Health Benefits of Narrative." *Literature and Medicine*, vol. 19, no. 1, 2000, pp. 3–18.

Refaie, Elizabeth El. *Autobiographical Comics: Life Writing in Pictures*. University Press of Mississippi, 2012.

Refaie, Elizabeth El. "Looking on the Dark and Bright Side: Creative Metaphors of Depression in Two Graphic Memoirs." *Auto/Biography Studies*, vol. 29, no. 1, 2014, pp. 149–174.

Sayce, Liz. *From Psychiatric Patient to Citizen*. Macmillan, 2000.

Scarry, Elaine. *The Body in Pain: The Making and Unmaking of the World*. Oxford UP, 1985.

Shivack, Nadia. *Inside Out: Portrait of an Eating Disorder*. Athenum Books for Young Readers, 2007.

Siegel, Linda. "The Use of Mural and Metaphor with a Schizophrenic Population for Recovery in a Trauma Situation." *Pratt Institute Creative Arts Therapy Review*, vol. 9, 1988, pp. 40–53.

Sledge, William H. "The Therapist's Use of Metaphor." *International Journal of Psychoanalysis*, vol. 6, no. 1, 1977, pp. 13–130.

Smith, Dan. "The Anorexic as Zombie Witness: Illness and Recovery in Katie Green's *Lighter Than My Shadow*." *The Walking Med: Zombies and the Medical Image*, edited Servitje L and Vint S, Penn State UP, 2016, pp. 190–214.

Sontag, Susan. *Illness as Metaphor*. Penguin, 1978.

Squier, Susan Merrill. "Literature and Medicine, Future Tense: Making it Graphic." *Literature and Medicine*, vol. 27, no. 2, 2008, pp. 124–152.

Steele, Williams, and Cathy A Malchiodi. *Trauma-informed Practices with Children and Adolescents*. Routledge, 2012.

Toombs, S Kay. "Illness and the Paradigm of Lived Body." *Theoretical Medicine*, vol. 9, no. 2, 1988, pp. 201–226.

Venkatesan, Sathyaraj, and Anu Mary Peter. "Life Is a Game: Visual Metaphors in Brian Fies' *Mom's Cancer*." *Hektoen International: A Journal of Medical Humanities*, Fall 2015.

Warin, Megan. *Abject Relations: Everyday Worlds of Anorexia*. Rutgers UP, 2009.

White, Michael, and David Epston. *Narrative Means to Therapeutic Ends.* Royal New Zealand Foundation of the Blind, 2015.

Williams, Ian. "Comics and the Iconography of Illness." *Graphic Medicine Manifesto*, edited Czerwiec MK et al., Penn State UP, 2015, pp. 115–142.

Wilson, Susannah. "Anorexia and Its Metaphors." *Exchanges: The Interdisciplinary Research Journal*, vol. 3, no. 2, 2016, pp. 216–226.

Zimmerman, Jeffrey L, and Victoria C Dickerson. *If Problems Talked: Narrative Therapy in Action.* Guilford Press, 1996.

5   From Abjection to Anorexia

Eating Disorders and the Horrors of the Female Body

It was in the second half of the twentieth century that feminists like Kim Chernin, Susan Bordo, Marcia Millman, and Laura S. Brown gave a gendered spin to eating disorders by emphasizing the role of societal norms in the etiology of eating disorders. Feminist interest in discourses on anorexia led to scholarly investigations of the socio-cultural meanings of women's starvation as well as the subjective interpretations of disordered eating habits. While socio-cultural theories throw sufficient light on external triggers, such as the thin body ideal, gendered biocultural analyses could unload the common misinterpretations that fixed anorexia as the epitome of women's obsession with beauty. The critical attention from feminists on women's phenomenological experience of eating disorders unfurled a plethora of causative factors ranging from sexual violence to abjection. Following a similar line of thought, most graphic pathographies attempt to spin the analysis of eating disorders beyond the cultural framework by giving subtle references to the contributory role of certain core feminine experiences like menstruation. The negative impact of menarche and the traumatic effect of sexual abuse, for instance, are extremely disempowering experiences that can adversely affect the body image of female adolescents (Ata et al.; Voelker et al.). While the contributory role of low body image and body shaming has been addressed exhaustively in eating disorder research, the possibilities of extending those arguments using theories of abjection had never been adequately examined until 2010 when Megan Warin explored the relationship between anorexia and abjection. Therefore, by using the theoretical postulates of Warin and other theoreticians of varying importance, this chapter examines the indirect role played by abjection in aggravating the tendency for eating disorders in women. Primary graphic narratives that are considered for close reading include Ludovic Debeurme's *Lucille* (2006), Nadia Shivack's *Inside Out: Portrait of an Eating Disorder* (2007), Lesley Fairfield's *Tyranny* (2009), Karrie Fransman's *The House That Groaned* (2012), and Katie Green's *Lighter Than My Shadow* (2013). In addition, this chapter also seeks to understand how the medium of comics aids disempowered sufferers in depicting their otherwise indescribable experiences of abjection during the course of their eating disorders.

Feminist Perspectives on Eating Disorders

During a time when medical science promulgated the psychological explanation of eating disorders in women as a mere manifestation of their derailed psyche, it was feminist theories that laid bare the cultural roots of eating disorders in women. Accordingly, major feminist theorists like Chernin, Bruch, Orbach, and Bordo consider the culture of thinness as a critical reason for the predominance of eating disorders among women. Feminist theorists argued that "women's bodies are a locus of social control" and raised their voices against the "19th century male dominated medicine [which] created nosologies that marked women as deviant" (Brumberg 37). Necessarily, by relying heavily on the cultural theoretical model, feminist theorists were successful in exposing how women and girls suffering from eating disorders were made "hapless victims of an all-powerful medical profession" (Brumberg 37). As Warin notes, "feminist work has importantly highlighted patriarchy, power, and gender relations as causal factors in the development of anorexia" (ix).

While feminist cultural theorists of eating disorder focused on the effect of cultural forces on women's body, corporeal feminists went a step ahead to include the impact of cultural factors on women's psyche also. As Josephine Brian observes,

> drawing on psychoanalysts like Freud and Lacan and phenomenologists like Merleau-Ponty, corporeal feminists approach the question of 'body image' not (solely) in terms of the body-as-image (as feminist culturalists arguably do) but in terms of the body's (psychic) imaging through perception and through its sensations and affects. (139)

However, due to their heavy reliance on the Lacanian theory of "sexual difference as the ultimate ground of subjectivity, corporeal feminists, in fact, come no closer than feminist culturalists do in allowing for the affective specificity of anorexic embodiment" (Brian 139). Interestingly, the biocultural approach can effectively address a plethora of causative factors of eating disorders, especially anorexia, identified by the feminist theorists over a period of time and can create a holistic understanding of the "affective and sentient aspects of anorexic embodiment" (Brian 18).

Accordingly, the biocultural readings of the feminist perspectives of eating disorders foreground that there could be more reasons behind a woman's self-starvation other than achieving a particular beauty ideal. As Becky Thompson points out:

> [s]ome women [were] raised in families and communities in which thinness was not considered a criterion for beauty. Yet, they still developed eating problems. Other women were taught that women should be thin, but their eating problems were not primarily in reaction to this imperative. Their eating strategies began as logical solutions to problems rather than problems themselves as they tried to cope with a variety of traumas. (558)

Thompson has extended the prominent analysis of eating disorders by stating that eating disorders could also "begin as ways women cope with various traumas including sexual abuse, racism, classism, sexism, heterosexism, and poverty" (547). According to Lazarus and Folkman, coping refers to "the thoughts and behaviors that people engage in so as to manage, tolerate, or reduce internal or external demands that are appraised as exceeding an individual's resources" (141). This definition reiterates the fact that eating disorders can result from experiences that are traumatic, intolerable, and self-altering. Considering the gravitas of those negative experiences on females, it is possible to redefine feelings such as self-repulsion, intense disgust with one's body and self, and horror about one's distorted body image, as instances of abjection in a strictly non-Kristevan way using Warin's perspectives on anorexia and abjection.

Abjection: Origin, and Popular Definitions

The word abject originated from the Latin word *abicere* meaning to throw away. Abject as a term garnered theoretical heft and significance with the rise of post-structuralism. *The Oxford Reference* defines the theoretical term abject as:

> [t]hat which disturbs the self, by provoking either disgust, fear, loathing or repulsion. Belonging to the realm of the psychic, the abject is the excessive dimension of either a subject or an object

that cannot be assimilated. As such, it is simultaneously outside or beyond the subject and inside and of the subject. Our own bodily fluids are for the most part loathsome to us, but the intensity of that loathing owes precisely to the fact that they come from us.

The concept of abjection has been adapted and applied in a variety of cultural fields, including psychoanalysis, literary criticism, visual studies, arts, sociology, psychotherapy, and organizational studies. The concept of abjection was developed by Georges Bataille, a French intellectual and literary critic, in his essay 'Abjection and Miserable Forms' written in 1934 and published posthumously in 1970 in *Essais de sociologie*. With a thematic thrust on the devastative socio-political impact of Hitler's rise to power, Bataille's essay deploys the term abject to discuss how a part of the population was considered to be outcasts who were "represented from the outside with disgust as the dregs of the people, populace and gutter" (Bataille 9). For Bataille, abject defined the social marginalization that was pervasive during the 1930s.

Bataille's socio-political theorization of abject was indubitably eclipsed by Kristeva's psychoanalytic definition of abjection that emerged with the publication of *Powers of Horror*. While Bataille's focus was on social abjection, Kristeva used the term abject to define human reactions like horror or repulsion to the disruption of meaning caused by the loss of distinction between subject and object or between self and other. Kristeva's notion of abjection relies heavily on the Lacanian paradigm and is a process that "pre-figures the mirror-stage in the psychic development of an infant" (Arya 48). According to Kristeva, abjection is something which "disturbs identity, system, order [and] does not respect boundaries, systems [or] rules" (4). Some items that can elicit such reactions are corpses, feces, body fluids, and sewage. Kristeva identifies three broad categories of abjections: (1) to food (2) to bodily waste, and (3) to sexual difference. In relation to bodily waste, leaky, squalid, and infected bodies are unapologetically ostracized from society for disrupting the notions of normalcy and for evoking disgust in others. It is essential at this point to note that this chapter is not concerned with the Kristevan psychoanalytic logic of abjection, rather it attempts to offer a different perspective of abjection in the context of eating disorders. To this end, this book draws on feminist perspectives of eating disorders as well as abject theory, particularly the theoretical postulates of Warin, to discuss how the tendency for anorexia in adolescent girls is aggravated by abjection due to menstruation.

**Abjection and Anorexia: Theoretical Interventions
of Megan Warin**

Before introducing Warin's adaptation of abject theory in anorexia studies anchored on disgust, it is essential to understand that this chapter does not use the term abject as a another sophisticated synonym for disgust; it is used as a term to qualify the utterly negative phenomenological experiences of female anorexics. From Kristeva's explanation of abjection as a feeling of repulsion, it is evident that disgust and fear are two terms on which the theory of abjection is positioned. Defining abjection as "the darkness that reigns at the heart of the human condition," Rina Arya, an acclaimed art theorist, argues that the Kristevan notion of abjection "highlights the ambivalent nature of disgust" (59). In her exploration of the theoretical convergence between disgust and abject, she observes that:

> the phenomenology of abjection bears similarities to the phenomenology of disgust in that both involve aversion to and rejection of a source that gives rise to feelings of repulsion. Throughout *Powers of Horror,* Kristeva theorises abjection in phenomenological terms associating it with bodily experiences (fluids, processes, and affects). Her archetypal example of abjection as the rejection of skin on milk can be used to show how the stages of behaviour mirror those experienced in disgust. (55)

Although disgust and abjection exist as individual theoretical corpuses, it is interesting to note that, while there are common characteristics like repulsion present in both abjection and disgust, it is the varying "degree of fear" (Arya 59) that makes disgust an instance of abjection. Though abjection "features as a region on the spectrum of disgust," disgust coupled with fear elicits abjection. As Arya contends, "[t]he degree of fear means that not all cases of disgust are abject" (59). Explaining the glaring lack of any palimpsests of the theory of abjection and disgust theory, Arya observes that

> the omission of abjection in studies about disgust can be explained by the different guiding concerns and methods used, in particular the psychoanalytical framework of abjection vis-à-vis Kristeva is not of interest to evolutionary psychologists or analytic philosophers. (59)

With this introduction to abjection, Warin's application of abject theory in the context of eating disorders is made easier. Published in 2010, *Abject Relations: Everyday Worlds of Anorexia* is the result of Warin's attempt to create "an alternative understanding of anorexia, one that will help make sense of the complexities of anorexia" (x). Although the book is moored on abject theory, Warin does not rely on the Kristevan psychoanalytic theory. Instead, she has extended the Kristevan concept of abject and attempted to give it an ethnographic grounding using the theory of relatedness. Defending her authorial motives, Warin notes that "[a]bjection, as I use it, moves beyond Kristeva's location of it in the imaginary, psyche, and language to the everyday practices and terms of sociality" (5). She further adds that the Kristevan concept of abject has

striking resonances with [her] field-work. Experiences of anorexia, like abjection, are fundamentally embodied, ambiguous, and transformative. While these terms —'embodiment,' 'ambiguity,' and 'transformation'— are themselves not abject, they are rendered abject in anorexia. (Warin 115)

Thus, by bringing the concepts of relatedness and abjection together into the analytical arena, this book raises new questions and new perspectives concerning not only anorexia but also the lives of those who are given this diagnosis. Warin's theoretical intervention offers particularly refreshing insights into the phenomenological experience of anorexia. It also reminds us that, despite the abundance of narratives about unbearable disgust, fear, exclusion, regression, and self-imposed exile from society experienced by anorexics, the causes of eating disorders have never been addressed using the concepts of abjection.

According to Warin:

[a]bjection play a central role in people's experiences of anorexia. This role was not deployed simply through language, but practiced through gendered bodies; the simultaneous hungering for and spitting out of foods; the physical retching of vomiting and purging; the erasure of sexual difference; the protection of bodies from contamination; elaborate cleansing routines (both internally and on the margins of bodies); and the desire to be clean, empty, and pure. (116)

Warin explores different ways in which women anorexics experienced physical feelings of repulsion, disgust, and horror about their bodies and certain bodily processes like menstruation, sexual abuse, sex, and pregnancy that she defines as "dangers associated with being female (implicitly female sexuality)" that are "construed as disgusting and too close for comfort" (17). Describing how the participants in her study described those experiences, Warin recollects that "they felt their bodies, like food, to be 'out of place,' 'dirty and polluted,' 'dangerous,' 'disgusting,' 'diseased,' 'contaminated,' 'soiled,' and 'impregnated with evil' . . . [and] these women experienced their bodies as inherently abject" (137). Anchored firmly on the popular notion of disgust which is "to be fully, indeed physically, conscious of being within the realm of uneasy categories . . . [that] causes the body to hide, to run away from its own cringing self" (Probyn 131–132), Warin's concept of anorexia as a corollary of abjection throws light on the significant role played by abjection caused by menstrual blood and traumatic memories of sexual abuse. Warin's *Abject Relations* gives a new dimension to the need for women anorexics "to protect themselves, clean themselves, and physically disappear" as a result of abjection (17). By essentially shifting the Kristevan "location of abjection beyond the symbolic, imaginary, psyche, and language" to "the interplay of senses that is central to this embodied abjection" (117), Warin offers an elaborate discussion of how "abjection pertains not only to foods, but also to gendered experiences (including events, places, and memories)" (17).

Menstrual blood is often referred to in theoretical contexts as an abject fluid (Freyja 8), and the menstruating body has served as a topic for feminist exploration of the systematic gendered governing of bodies. Extending the theory of abject beyond the psychoanalytical framework to disgust and stigma, Imogen Tyler ("Social Abjection") observes in his notes on social stigma: "[t]he abject is a concept which describes all that is repulsive and fascinating about bodies and in particular those aspects of bodily experience which unsettle bodily integrity: death, decay, fluids, orifices, sex, defecation, vomiting, illness, menstruation, pregnancy and childbirth." According to Kristeva, bodily fluids are defined as "'flow, discharge, haemorrhage' which threatens to engulf us" (5). In her seminal work, *The Woman in the Body*, Emily Martin suggests that the feminine body-perception has been influenced phenomenally by "the language and models of medical discourse that has created an overwhelmingly negative interpretation of their bodily experiences like menstruation, childbirth, and menopause" (qtd. in Warin 136). She argues that scientific models denigrate women's bodily experiences by describing such experiences using terms implying failed production, waste, decay, and breakdown. Menstruation, for example, is described in standard texts for medical students as a negative process, exemplified by words such as "failure," "deprivation," "constriction," "diminished," "disintegration," "hemorrhage," "debris," "loss," and "necrosis"" (Warin 197). Although menstruation has long been posited at the socio-cultural crossroads as a taboo experience, it received a renewed theoretical attention when bodily fluids gained centrality in Kristeva's concept of abjection.

While it is true that menstruation is not an essential aspect of eating disorder literature since anorexics do not menstruate, it has a significant role in the initiation of disordered eating habits in many adolescent girls. Many found that menarche and the less laudable bodily transformation it causes in a teenager enhance body dissatisfaction which can be an indirect reason for disordered eating patterns (Ata et al.; Huebscher). Attaining puberty later or earlier than peers can also affect body image as well as psychological health. According to Ata et al., girls tend to become vulnerable, sensitive, and self-conscious about their weight during the onset of menstruation, which will, in turn, affect their self-esteem. Girls who get picked on for being overweight or underweight could be driven into gaining or losing weight in an unhealthy way and research has found that there is a correlation between body image and self-esteem among early-adolescent age groups (Davison and McCabe). Theoretically, the disgust and fear that girls feel about their bodily transformations during puberty can be understood in terms of self-abjection (Lesnik-Oberstein). It is the impact of abjection that eating disorder sufferers attempt to manage using maladaptive coping strategies like restrictive eating. While cultural issues are systematically addressed in verbal narratives of eating disorders, one of the prominent aspects of women's eating disorders highlighted in graphic narratives is how abjection caused by the changes that occur in the female body during or after menarche could lead to eating disorders. Autobiographical graphic narratives like *Lighter* and *Tyranny* offer insights about abjection as a contributory factor of eating disorders.

"I Feel Disgusting": Menstruation and Abjection in *Lighter Than My Shadow*

Unlike other eating disorder narratives, Katie Green's *Lighter Than My Shadow* is a memoir that touches upon various issues that make anorexia nervosa a truly corporeal feminist concern. In addition to discussing Katie's experience of anorexia, binge,

Obsessive Compulsive Disorder (OCD), and Post-Traumatic Stress Disorder (PTSD), the graphic memoir also focuses on every minute incident that contributed to her disordered eating. One such incident that Green brings to the reader's attention is the disruptive impact of her first 'period' on Katie's body perception on the first day of secondary school. Katie's picky eating behavior aggravates into a full-blown condition of clinical anorexia as a result of the body shaming that she experiences in secondary school. Therefore, Katie's entry into secondary school is a crucial juncture in the narrative because of the tremendous negative impact it has on her body esteem. Unlike other girls her age, Katie was utterly ignorant of the fashion-conscious lifestyle that kids would flaunt in school. It was following a conversation with her friend Megan on the day before the first day at secondary school that Katie painfully realizes her lack of conformity with the rest of the girls and that she does not fit in (see Chapter 4 for more details). The harsh realization about her out-of-style dresses, accessories, and appearance shatters Katie's self-confidence to the extent that she believes herself to be unprepared for the school. She breaks into tears and throws herself into her mother's arms, repeatedly telling that she doesn't want to go to school (43). When her father enquires about the unusual fuss that Katie is making instead of leaving for school, she shouts "I'm not ready!" at him and goes inside.

Green's masterly use of facial expressions and gestures to communicate Katie's experience of abjection reiterates a quality unique to the medium of comics—economy of expression. While depicting the emotional disturbance that Katie experienced before going to school, Green provides a scene where readers see Katie as scrutinizing herself in front of a mirror. The mirror image gives the exact mapping of Katie's psychological turmoil through her eyes swelling up with tears, the intense self-doubting look, curved down lips, eyebrows raised in anxiety, messy hair, shoulders that are drooping down in shame, oversized uniform, and an incorrectly worn tie. When Katie is seen as psychologically struggling with an unutterable woe, Green refrains from verbally describing Katie's agony. Instead, Green makes use of gestures and body language to communicate Katie's pain. As Will Eisner contends, "body posture and gesture occupy a position of supremacy over text. The manner in which these images are employed modifies and defines the intended meaning of the words" (106).

Upon realizing that she has started menstruating, Katie becomes reticent and shrinks into herself with shame and uneasiness. When

Katie's mother tells about menstruation, one aspect of menstruation that startles Katie is that the menstrual blood might leak. As Brook reminds, menstruation is regarded across cultures as one of the "polluting or abject properties of adult female bodies" (50). When her mother says: "You'll need to change it every few hours and check it doesn't leak," Katie is seen as imagining the embarrassment it could bring to her in a public space (45). It is in a horizontal tier that is unsymmetrically segregated into two panels that Green depicts Katie's apprehensions about being a leaky body. Interestingly, the two images of Katie securely sitting in her bedroom with her mother and Katie standing alone in a public space with fingers being vehemently pointed at her also mediates the idea of social stigma around menstruating females. The adept use of emanatas in the image amplifies the impact of stigmatization on Katie. Functioning more as an inset that reflects Katie's mind, this panel could be seen as an instance of Green's experimentation with drawing styles. Irrespective of the fact that it is a thought balloon, Green has depicted it more as a panel in itself owing to the wealth of meanings that it carries. Katie's bewilderment in standing in a puddle of menstrual blood trickling down her legs is realistically conveyed through her posture and facial expression. Instead of assuming a lady like posture, Katie is depicted as standing with her legs apart, hands firmly folded in a self-defensive manner. The hands that are pointed towards Katie could be socio-cultural institutions like religion and society that consider menstruation as taboo. It is interesting to note that instead of using appropriate words such as blood and sanitary pad, Katie's mother uses the pronoun "it" to refer to the process and facilities related to menstruation. Her advice also emphasizes the social embarrassment that Katie would have to suffer if she doesn't change the sanitary pad every few hours to avoid leakage.

Katie's distress turns into disgust when she realizes that her menstrual blood can smell if she doesn't take baths twice a day. Katie gets confused and helpless trying to understand the sudden transformation of her otherwise normal body to that of a leaky and stinky one. The onset of menstruation forces Katie towards developing a strong sense of self-abjection and hatred towards her feminine body. Reiterating Elizabeth Grozs' observations, Green depicts

> the ways that the menstrual markers of a young woman's puberty are enmeshed in a signification of stains, loss of control, and leakage which draws her back into the dependency and

inadequacy of infancy rather than forward into self-contained adulthood: 'the impulsion into a future of a past that she thought she had left behind'. (205)

Thus, Green gives a graphic representation of how menstrual blood is considered as a defiling bodily fluid (Kristeva) and how menstruating females are culturally understood as abject women without any control over their bodily functions.

Katie's feeling of being a personification of abjection aggrandizes as she leaves the secureness of her home for school which was "bad enough already" (48). Katie expresses her overpowering sense of abjection in being a menstruating body by keeping her head hung in shame and disgust all through the day. On the way, she confesses her current state to her friend by saying: "I feel disgusting" (46). The fact that her friend has not started menstruating makes Katie chagrined. When Megan asks Katie to describe what is menstruation on their way to school, Katie embarrassingly reveals: "Er . . . like blood" (46). Megan instantly expresses her repulsion by characterizing menstruation as something "[g]ross" (46). Green once again deploys facial expressions like a wrinkled nose and widely opened eyes to convey Megan's mixed feelings of disgust and astonishment. Megan also unnerves Katie by bringing up the issue of leakage. When Katie says that the menstrual blood will leak out and she has to keep checking, Megan gives a humiliating sound characteristic of repulsion, "Eww!", together with a sardonic grin (46). Additionally, Megan mentions the popular conception of menstruation as a perilous corporeal condition. Megan unapologetically tells Katie that tall girls will menstruate early and therefore she is "safe for a few more years" when compared to Katie (47). This worsens Katie's inner turmoil to the extent that she considers herself an ill-fated girl. Upon realizing that Megan's aversion has increased manifold, Katie's helplessness and shame transform into an extreme state of self-abjection which forces her to confess: "I feel disgusting" (46). Indubitably, Katie's self-denigration lucidly underscores the impact of menstruation as a condition of abjection on girls.

Unsurprisingly, the discomfort in being in her skin increases double-fold when she reaches the school. Alleviating Katie's problematic misunderstanding of her body and self as disgusting, she gets body shamed by three boys in her school. They heckle, humiliate, and trip her in the school corridor. Calling Katie by the name 'Neil' (48), they successfully accentuate her self-disgust. Afraid of further humiliation, and unable to bear the heft of shame and helplessness, Katie flees to the girl's toilet, where she is astounded to see girls thronging in the common area, enthusiastically engaged in putting on make-up, or combing. Using three consecutive panels, Green adeptly communicates Katie's notion of being a misfit among other girls her age. The first tier essentially functions as a visual attestation of how Katie, as an abject and misfit, is ostracized from the society. While Katie stands teary eyed wearing an oversized uniform at the door step, Green is allowing a comparison of Katie with other stylish girls in mini-skirt model uniforms. Katie wades through the crowd and hides in the toilet. Katie's posture sums up the magnitude of her feelings of abjection and embarrassment caused by menstruation and body shaming. Towards the middle of the narrative, Katie assumes the same posture at her therapist's home during a moment of intense trauma followed by an incident of sexual abuse.

Katie gets body shamed multiple times within and outside of the school for her lack of feminine beauty, often exemplified through hair-free hands and legs, stylized hair, fashionable dress, and accessories. On another day, the same boys harass Katie on her way to school. They humiliate her for not having her legs waxed like other girls. Predominantly in western culture, body hair in women is a mark of undesirability as "the hairless female body also functions as a measure of feminine attractiveness" (Lesnik-Oberstein 70). From Katie's experience, it is clear that the "cultural hostility to 'superfluous' female hair can perhaps be understood in terms of Mary Douglas's theory of pollution and Julia Kristeva's concept of abjection" (Lesnik-Oberstein 69). While Katie tries to walk away without retaliating, they snatch her school bag, take out a sanitary pad, and flaunt it. Green makes it clear to readers that Katie was terrified about leaks, foul smell, and essentially about being a repulsive body because she understood menstruation as a disgustful condition of awkwardness, dishonor, and "an arbitrary stroke of very bad luck" (Carel 37). While Katie was in an urgency to hide from the rest of the world, she wanted to guard the secrecy around her menstruation by not exhibiting sanitary pads or allowing herself to be stained. Therefore, the incident in which the boys expose Katie's feminine secret traumatizes her. For Katie, whose self-confidence was walloped by Megan on the previous day and worsened by the onset of menstruation, body shaming on the very first day of secondary school turns out to be detrimental. After this incident, Katie starts exhibiting disordered eating patterns and she eventually resorts to extreme dieting and attains an enviable body shape; however, she becomes an anorexic. Katie's experience of body shaming and self-disgust graphically reiterates Brook's observation that the onset of menstruation is "[t]he marker of female adulthood with its accompanying dangerous entry into the abject" (51).

One of the interesting formal experiments that Green has deployed in the memoir is the incredibly creative use of various color tones. According to Jan Beatens, "colour is undoubtedly one of the most underdiscussed and undertheorized features of comics and graphic novel scholarship" (111). Deviating slightly from the monochromatic grey tones used in the earlier pages, Green has used a subtle shade of pale purple in the pages that contain the conversation about menstruation. While black, white, and grey remain the predominant shades, the occasional shift to pastel shades and variants of mauve in selected pages exemplifies the emotional significance of certain incidents in the narrative. Although it is difficult to trace the meaning of each background shade that is used by the memoirist, the colors definitely enhance the experience of reading by adding "context to events or to her moods and feelings" (Leblanc n.p).

"I Hate This. I Hate Me": Menstruation and Abjection in *Tyranny*

A strikingly similar instance is available in Lesley Fairfield's *Tyranny*, one of the earliest graphic narratives to talk about the complex interface between menstruation and abjection in an anorexic's life. *Tyranny* describes the experience of self-disgust that Anna, the protagonist, experiences with the onset of menstruation. Fairfield brings up the topic of menstruation on the third page of the memoir. Defining the day when she got her first period as the critical juncture when "things began to change" (7), Fairfield thereafter dedicates five pages to elaborate upon the impact of menstruation on Anna's body as well as her life. Anna mistakes her bodily transformations during maturation as weight gain and believes that periods made her body bigger. A false body perception infiltrates her mind, and she develops hatred towards her body that grew out-of-proportion over a period of time after she began menstruating. Even though Anna's mother tries to console her by saying: "You're not too big!. . . This is all a very normal part of growing up," Anna mourns: "[b]ut it looks like fat to me, mom" (9). Mom attempts to pacify Anna by saying: "well it's not, dear. Just be careful you don't gain too much more weight" (9).

Another significant change that happens in Anna's life at that time is that her father stops hugging her. Anna confesses that she misunderstood him when he justified: "I'm just trying to give you space, honey" (9). Anna felt like she lost her body after menstruating and what she had was a fat and ugly body. She reminiscences with shock: "I felt trapped inside my new body!" (10). Unable to handle the desperation and self-repulsion, Anna takes her mother's advice seriously and believes that her "new body" could be controlled through starvation and dieting in order to regain her "younger body back" (10). She decides to diet and eventually becomes anorexic.

Fairfield's strategic use of the comicscape to convey Anna's feeling of self-abjection is remarkable. For the first time, readers see an expression of perplexity on Anna's face when she gets her first period. It is when Anna gets her first period that readers see Fairfield's experimentation with panel borders to communicate the notion of excess and transgression. According to Douglas, "menstruation is, like childbirth, a liminal and therefore abject condition where the female body is perceived (by men) as changing shape and transgressing from the 'natural' human state whereby blood and other bodily fluids are contained" (qtd. in Brook 51). Anna's experience and firm belief that her body underwent some change with her first period is visually hinted by depicting Anna's buttock outside the panel framework. Similarly, in the next page when Anna and her mother go shopping for undergarments, Anna is seen as stunned at seeing her gigantic and out of proportional mirror image. Anna's reflection is depicted as too big to be contained within the existing panels, therefore conveying the notion of enormousness and transcendence, and her breasts are pictured as ballooning out of the panel. As Beatens notes:

> [t]he frames are no longer a passive reinforcement of the structure of the panels, but an active player in the ecosystem of the comic strip where it actively intervenes so that a rupture at the level of the drawings can be compensated by a new device at a higher level. (126)

The idea of disgust and abjection gets graphically manifested in the following splash page where Anna is seen as engaged in a symbolic struggle with her voluptuous selves. Fairfield depicts Anna's sense of abjection by drawing a multitude of naked, euphoric, and fat versions of Anna climbing on her body, pulling her hair, and driving her crazy. Anna confesses: "My imagination worked over time, and before long I was tormented and miserable" (10). Anna's experience of desperation, helplessness, and self-abjection are effectively portrayed through the image of her being overpowered by her own naked selves while she mutters in a frenzy: "I hate this. I hate me" (10). Standing amidst the chaos created by her miniatures, Anna is seen as shouting: "Let me out" (11). Anna's psychological mayhem alleviates only when she starts dieting. Soon she attains a self-realization that slenderness is perfection and happiness. Anna is depicted in another splash page as standing on top of the world in larger than life size, shouting "As long as I'm thin and perfect, I'll be invincible" (16–17). Fairfield also subtly hints at the impact of advertisements and popular culture through the sticker which reads, "Mirrors Don't Lie" placed in the dressing room.

Similar instances are also available in Ludovic Debeurme's *Lucille*, Nadia Shivack's *Inside Out: Portrait of an Eating Disorder*, and Karrie Fransman's *The House That Groaned*. Through a fictional graphic narrative, *Lucille* discusses the life of Lucille, a girl who becomes anorexic as a result of increased self-disgust. Commenting on her childhood, Lucille recollects that she was a chubby little girl who had a special bond with her father. However, Lucille's relationship with her parents as well as with herself was destroyed after she witnessed her father and mother engaged in sexual intercourse. Calling it a "violent" experience that damaged her life forever, Lucille reminisces: "Odd . . . Ever since my weight dropped" (n.p.). Another incident that aggravated her self-esteem was realizing that no boy is interested in girls who are "chubby" (n.p.). While playing a ball game in the lake with some friends in the summer, Lucille was startled and ashamed to find that the boys would never aim at her because she was fat and ugly compared to other girls who were slender and beautiful. Deburme depicts Lucille's height of shame and aversion through the image of Lucille trying to hide from the world by drowning herself in the water. Lucille confesses thus to the readers: "[t]hat was when I realised that the ball would never hit me. . . [so] I wanted to hide myself completely from view."

In due course of time, Lucille's disgust developed into an overwhelming feeling of abjection, and she yearned to be invisible by growing frail. Lucille's sense of abjection is manifest when she says "food fills me up. It's heaviness in my stomach disgusts me" (n.p.). As a consequence of her abjecthood, Lucille believes that she looks like "crap" and develops disordered eating behavior (n.p.). In a strikingly similar vein, Janet in Fransman's *The House That Groaned* becomes anorexic after catching her husband Adam having sex with his male friend. In her memoir, *Inside Out: Portrait of an Eating Disorder* published in 2007, Nadia Shivack also offers insights into the complex association between abjecthood and eating disorder. About the role of binging and purging in plummeting Nad's self-esteem, Shivack notes: "[e]verything about me is 'small' now except for the shame and despair" and she perceives herself as a "greedy girl" with a "full, fat, [and] filthy" stomach (n.p.). In essence, these graphic narratives on eating disorders offer insights about eating disorders in women as a consequence of disgust and abjection. Using the formal features of the medium of comics, graphic medicine depicts how "abjection pertains not only to foods, but also to gendered experiences (including events, places, and memories)" (Warin 17).

"I'm Disgusting": Self-Disgust and Sexual Abuse

Disgust, as maintained by Menninghaus, is a "state of alarm and emergency, an acute crisis of self-preservation in the face of an unassimilable otherness, a convulsive struggle, in which what is in question is, quite literally, whether 'to be or not to be'" (1). Identified as a rejection response to events, things, persons, or experiences that could be triggered through smell, touch, vision, or intellect, disgust always affects "the whole nervous system" (Menninghaus 1). According to Feldner et al. (12), sexual abuse is one of the traumatic events that could stimulate disgust towards oneself. Various research studies document that female victims of sexual abuse are likely to experience intense urges to clean themselves because of an overriding feeling of being dirty (de Silva and Marks 1999; Gershuny et al. 2003; Fairbrother and Rachman 2004). Commenting on the disgust and abjection in *Abject Relations*, Warin observes that

> [d]isgust is the core sensation on which abjection turns. When disgust comes too close, as in being raped or imbibing dirty food, the body is violated and needs to be distanced. Distancing means reducing it, disconnecting experiences, cleaning it, and numbing it. (139)

Menninghaus agrees with this notion when he contends that "Kristeva's description of abjection, from the beginning, suggests an affinity with disgust" (373). In the case of females with eating disorders, sexual abuse is often found to be a stimulant that aggravates their sense of abjection and disgust towards their leaky and out of control bodies.

In *Lighter Than My Shadow*, Green exemplifies how sexual abuse along with a plethora of factors such as menstruation, low self-esteem, and body shaming has "coalesced to form an embodied sense of disgust" (Warin 140) that eventually transmutes to eating disorders in Katie. In an interview given to Diana Denza for National Eating Disorder Association, Katie Green recollects that the most challenging process during the creation of *Lighter Than My Shadow* was drawing the scenes of sexual abuse. In a similar vein, talking to Karen Walsh in an interview given in NYCC in 2018, Green noted that sexual abuse in the context of eating disorders is never sufficiently addressed. Speaking on the impact of sexual abuse, Green again recollects: "I would draw a tiny panel, and then cover it up with a piece of paper so I didn't have to look at it while I drew the next piece because it was just horrible" (Walsh n.p). While Green's words accurately reflect her fear, they also underscore the feeling of disgust that she felt about her recovery, and Green's depictions of Katie before and after the sexual abuse effectively communicates the same.

After repeated body shaming at school, as well as other reasons, Katie is clinically diagnosed as anorexic. However, Katie resorts to alternate therapy with Jake, the therapist who claimed to "work with stuck energy in the body" (228). Jake persuades Katie to believe that the key to her recovery from anorexia lies in her independence and absolute freedom from her parents' control. With regard to Jake and his support, Katie explains: "He's given me so much confidence to stand up for myself, break away from my family. They drain my energy. They're part of why I got sick" (286). During therapy sessions, Jake repeatedly tells Katie: "leaving home is going to be the best thing you've ever done. You'll discover how strong you are. You'll shine" (p. 241). Katie slowly becomes convinced that Jake's place is much safer and better compared to her home. Jake effortlessly wins Katie's trust by offering much needed appreciation and acknowledgement that she rarely received from her family. With Jake's help, Katie eventually made others believe that she had recovered as she gained a sense of control over herself. Under Jake's magical influence, Katie compromised her family, her best friend Megan, and her long-term boyfriend, Ed. Once Katie was cut off from them, she was invited to attend a summer festival with Jake and his family, and she was sexually abused by Jake. Utterly devastated by the incident, Katie absconds and consequently develops enormous disgust towards herself for trusting "a brainwashing psycho" (312), and for allowing him to taint her sense of purity. As a cumulative impact of the feeling of abjection, disgust, and fear, Katie starts binge eating.

Although Green sticks to the conventional panel structure, she introduces at various points other shades like violet and subtle shades of green. Using a purple hair dye, Green manages to communicate the positive feeling or transformation that Katie experienced after meeting Jake. While her body structure remains the same, the hair color acts as the marker of an enchanting phase in Katie's journey. When the pages that describe the events that happened leading up to the sexual abuse are doused in a beautiful pastel shade of pink symbolic of Katie's adolescence and joy, the episode of sexual assault is depicted against a dull shade of green. Followed by the depiction of the harrowing incident, the color tone shifts back to the various shades of grey. Green's evocative and powerful drawings of Katie's sexual assault exemplify the ability of the medium of comics to articulate emotions that are too intense to be communicated through words using eyes, eyebrows, lips, and jaws. Green deploys a range of gestures and facial expressions while narrating the episode of sexual abuse. In order to trace the sudden shifts in Katie's emotions from enchantment to shock, shock to anger, anger into horror which culminates in helplessness, Green uses only the eyebrows and lips. Suggestive of how the physical assault was going to be the most harrowing experience in Katie's struggle towards recovery, the panels are given a vignette effect with the thick patch of darkness as a visual metaphor of the agonizing impact of body shaming on Katie that happened in secondary school. As the thick patch of darkness encroaches into the frame, Green zooms further into the scene, allowing readers to experience Katie's trauma as Jake advances towards her.

Accurately expressing the intensity of her pain and horror, the very next page has a full-page panel that depicts the sexual abuse in detail using incomplete flashes of images. The panel filled with darkness represents Katie's mind that was flooded with memories of body shaming and horror. Although Katie runs out of Jake's tent, she feels as though she is being chased by him into the jungle. The image of the abuser's hand emerging out of the pitch-black darkness towards Katie as she runs away captures her mental doldrum. Green uses emanatas to show Katie trembling with fear on seeing Jake's smiling face all around her. Thereafter, Katie is seen as sitting under a tree, huddled to herself, and pulling her hair in disgust just the way she sat in the secondary school toilet after getting body shamed on the first day. Katie breaks down into tears while muttering in disbelief and disgust: "I'm so stupid. . . How could I be so stupid?" (313). Katie's expressions of trauma reiterate the detrimental impact of physical violation from a trusted person. Apart from physical assault, Katie's trust was also destroyed at multiple levels. After a point in time, Katie loses her faith in Jake, whom she believed more than herself. Katie invested so much in trusting Jake, believing that he was the only person who could understand her body issues and help her. She was ready to believe that she had recovered "if Jake said so" (251). After the incident, Katie realizes that her mother and Megan were right about him, and that he never wanted to help her. Such a realization forced Katie to accept that her recovery from anorexia was a lie that Jake created to win her trust. In a panel that is filling up with darkness emerging out of Katie's broken head is an adept picturization of her statement: "My whole recovery is based on this . . . on him" (313). Soon she is depicted as breaking into pieces and dissolving into the patch of darkness, suggesting how her sense of self itself was destroyed by Jake. Unable to believe that she was sexually abused by Jake, Katie tries to convince herself that such an incident never happened, and she keeps it a secret from everyone else.

According to Goldner-Vukov and Moore, apart from "logically making sense of trauma, the survivor has to cope with profound emotional problems of guilt, shame, resentment, hatred, vengeance as well as forgiveness and reconciliation" (3). Binging provided Katie a temporary sense of relief from being out of control, but the satisfaction never lasted long. To regain control over her body that was lost during the abuse, Katie tries to avoid eating. However, she starts losing her self-control and binges during the night. Surprisingly, Katie resorts to food and eating as a way of coping with the distress. Katie's binge eating is symbolically represented through the image of an agape mouth filled with the symbolic pitch-black darkness on her stomach. Even though Katie wanted to stop binge eating, she never succeeded. Eventually, Katie develops self-hatred for her uncontrolled eating.

Regarding her out of control eating, Katie states in an apologetic manner: "[t]he more I binged, the more I punished myself . . . can't believe I kep[t] on doing it. I'm so disgusting" (342). To bring it under control, Katie restricted her eating to some extent and continued her exercises. But she badly failed in controlling the tendency to binge, and Katie's feeling of self-abjection kept increasing after every episode of binging. As she recollects: "[t]he relief only lasted a moment . . . then came the guilt and disgust" (372). While dumping all the food items into the trash bin to avoid binging, Katie is seen as scolding herself: "Why do I keep being disgusting? Can't believe I'm so disgusting" (351). Unfortunately, Katie's craving for control forces her to devour more food, and Green gives a sad graphic presentation of Katie eating food from the trash bin.

Katie's disgust towards her body self magnifies and makes her believe that she is contaminated and impure. Katie's transformation into a self-defined abject body is evident when she laments: "I was clean, pure, in control. Now I can never go back. I'm disgusting [and] this is all I deserve" (373). As Warin contends, women with eating disorders:

> often use similar repulsive metaphors to explain their experiences, describing themselves as like "toilets," "full of shit," "garbage," "scum," and "rubbish." They felt their bodies, like food, to be "out of place," "dirty and polluted," "dangerous," "disgusting," "diseased," "contaminated," "soiled," and "impregnated with evil." More than Martin's metaphors of "failed production," these women experienced their bodies as inherently abject. (137)

Considering her body as a corporeal remnant of disgust and guilt, Katie even imagines chiseling away her flesh, and decides to commit suicide. However, towards the end of the narrative, Katie makes peace with her past and starts feeling positive about her body through art therapy, counseling, and care. Reiterating Warin's observations, *Lighter* is a graphic expression of Green's "attempt to create boundaries and effect closure or, in other words, to defeat abjection" (17).

Conclusion

Unpacking the popular notions of eating disorders as "the epitome of a Western obsession with individualism, self- control, and autonomy," this chapter has examined various ways in which girls experience their bodies as abject, disgusting, and impure due to body shaming during menstruation (Warin 2). Katie in Green's *Lighter Than My Shadow*, Lucille in Debeurme's *Lucille*, Nad in Shivack's *Inside Out: Portrait of an Eating Disorder*, Anna in Fairfield's *Tyranny*, and Janet in Fransman's *The House That Groaned* are powerful examples of how women suffering from eating disorders deploy body as a medium to communicate their ineffable emotions related to body shaming and abjection primarily through gestures. By close reading select graphic medicine narratives, this chapter has examined various ways in which girls have experienced their bodies as abject, disgusting, and impure due to sexual abuse or body shaming and menstruation. Since the emotional scars from such incidents further precipitate the aversion to their body and self, women would indulge in self-starvation or binging while trying to manage the shame, and thereby to resolve the derailed relationship with their bodies. Gendered analyses of eating disorders thus help to reconfigure the existing notions of eating disorder as a cultural problem that happens to women who are obsessed with body perfection and fashion. In essence, an attempt is made to rescript eating disorders in women as a corollary of abjection that is "utterly continuous with a dominant element of the experience of being female in this culture" (Bordo 57).

Works Cited

Arya, Rina. "Abjection Interrogated Uncovering the Relation between Abjection and Disgust." *Journal of Extreme Anthropology*, vol. 1, no.1. 2017, pp. 48–61.

Ata, Rheanna N et al. "The Effects of Gender and Family, Friend, and Media Influences on Eating Behaviors and Body Image during Adolescence." *Journal of Youth and Adolescence*, vol. 36, no. 8, 2006, pp. 1024–1037.

Baetens, Jan. "From Black & White to Color and Back: What Does It Mean (Not) to Use Color?" *College Literature*, vol. 38, no. 3, 2011, pp. 111–128.

Bataille, Georges. "'L'Abjection et les formes misérables.'" *Essais de sociologie Œuvrescomplètes*, vol. 2, 1970, pp. 217–221.

Bordo, Susan. *Unbearable Weight: Feminism, Western Culture, and the Body*. U of California P, 2004.

Brian, Josephine. *Hungry for Meaning: Discourses of the Anorexic Body*. Diss. London School of Economics and Political Science (United Kingdom), 2006.

Brook, Barabara. *Feminist Perspectives on the Body*. Routledge, 2014.

Brumberg, Joan Jacobs. *Fasting Girls: The History of Anorexia Nervosa*. Vintage Books, 2000.

Carel, Havi. *Illness: The Cry of the Flesh*. Routledge, 2013.

Davison, Tanya E, and Marita P McCabe. "Adolescent Body Image and Psychosocial Functioning." *The Journal of Social Psychology*, vol. 146, 2006, pp. 15–30.

Debeurme, Ludovic. *Lucille*. Top Shelf Productions, 2011.

de Silva, Padmal, and Melanie Marks. "The Role of Traumatic Experiences in the Genesis of Obsessive–Compulsive Disorder." *Behaviour Research and Therapy*, vol. 37, no. 10, 1999, pp. 941–951.

Eisner, Will. *Comics and Sequential Art: Principles and Practices from the Legendary Cartoonist*. W.W. Norton, 2008.

Fairbrother, Nichole, and S Rachman. "Feelings of Mental Pollution Subsequent to Sexual Assault." *Behaviour Research and Therapy*, vol. 42, no. 2, 2004, pp. 173–189.

Fairfield, Lesley. *Tyranny*. Tundra Books, 2009.

Feldner, Matthew T et al. "An Empirical Test of the Association between Disgust and Sexual Assault." *International Journal of Cognitive Therapy*, vol. 3, no. 1, 2010, pp. 11–22.

Freyja Jónudóttir, Barkardóttir. *Hope of Failure: Subverting Disgust, Shame and the Abject in Feminist Performances with Menstrual Blood*. 2016, Utrecht University, Master dissertation. *Utrecht University Repository*, https://dspace.library.uu.nl/handle/1874/338547. Accessed 23 May 2018.

Gershuny, Beth S et al. "Comorbid Posttraumatic Stress Disorder: Impact on Treatment Outcome for Obsessive-Compulsive Disorder." *American Journal of Psychiatry*, vol. 159, no. 5, 2002, pp. 852–854.

Goldner-Vukov, Mila, and Laurie Jo Moore. "The Meaning of Sexual Abuse." *Journal of Psychology & Psychotherapy*, vol. 1, 2011, p. 101.

Green, Katie. "*Lighter Than My Shadow*." Interview by Diana Denza. *National Eating Disorder Association*, www.nationaleatingdisorders.org/blog/lighter-than-my-shadow-memoir-katie-green-interview. Accessed 23 Jan. 2019.

Green, Katie. *Lighter Than My Shadow*. Random House, 2013.

Green, Katie. "NYCC 2018: Katie Green from Lion Forge-'*Lighter Than My Shadow*.'" Interview by Karen Walsh. *Geek Mom*, 18 Oct. 2018, https://geekmom.com/2018/10/nycc-2018-katie-green-from-lion-forge-lighter-than-my-shadow/. Accessed 23 Jan. 2019.

Huebscher, Brenda. *Relationship between Body Image and Self-Esteem among Adolescent Girls*. 2010. U of Wisconsin-Stout, PhD dissertation.

Kristeva, Julia et al. "Cultural Crossings of Care: An Appeal to the Medical Humanities." *Medical Humanities*, vol. 44, no. 1, 2018, pp. 55–58.

Lazarus, Richard S, and Susan Folkman. *Stress, Appraisal, and Coping*. Springer, 1984.

Leblanc, Philippe. "*Lighter Than My Shadow* or Katie Green's Masterpiece." *The Beat*, 29 Mar. 2018, www.comicsbeat.com/review-lighter-than-my-shadow/. Accessed 12 May 2019.

Lesnik-Oberstein, Karín. *The Last Taboo: Women and Body Hair*. Manchester UP, 2006.

Martin, Emily. *The Woman in the Body: A Cultural Analysis of Reproduction*. Beacon Press, 2003.

Menninghaus, Winfried. *Disgust: The Theory and History of a Strong Sensation.* State U of New York P, 2003.

O'Connor, Richard A, and Esterik P Van. "De-medicalizing Anorexia: A New Cultural Brokering." *Anthropology Today*, vol. 24, no. 5, 2008, pp. 6–9.

Probyn, Elizabeth. "The Anorexic Body." *Body Invaders, Panic Sex in America*, edited Kroker A and Kroker M, New World Perspectives, CultureTexts Series, Oxford UP, 1987.

Shivack, Nadia. *Inside Out: Portrait of an Eating Disorder.* Athenum Books for Young Readers, 2007.

Thompson, Becky W. ""A Way Outa No Way": Eating Problems among African-American, Latina, and White Women." *Gender and Society*, vol. 6, no. 4, 1992, pp. 546–561.

Tyler, Imogen. *Revolting Subjects: Social Abjection and Resistance in Neoliberal Britain.* Zed Books Ltd., 2013.

Voelker, Dana K et al. "Weight Status and Body Image Perceptions in Adolescents: Current Perspectives." *Adolescent Health, Medicine and Therapeutics*, vol. 6, 2015, pp. 149–158.

Warin, Megan. *Abject Relations: Everyday Worlds of Anorexia.* Rutgers UP, 2009.

Conclusion
Towards an Alternative
Understanding of Eating Disorders

Practiced as a form of religious sacrifice in the twelfth century, and been identified thereafter as a defensive mode of self-starvation, and construed later in the Victorian era as an exclusive feminine malady, eating disorders have never been a part of social discussions in the initial days. Although the earliest medical descriptions of anorexia were brought out in 1689 through Richard Morton's *Phthisiologia, Or, A Treatise of Consumptions*, it took another century for medical science to accept anorexia nervosa as an illness condition. However, eating disorders remained unfamiliar to common man for yet another century as dialogues on eating disorders were constrained within the limits of psychiatry until Bruch's *The Golden Cage: The Enigma of Anorexia Nervosa* in 1978 was published. Following the intrepid steps of Bruch, many patients, clinicians, and thinkers contributed to the wealth of eating disorder literature through memoirs, autobiographical narratives, fictions, and theoretical findings, among others. While patients in the eighteenth and nineteenth centuries resorted solely to verbal medium to narrate their eating disorder experience, the post-millennial era turned to a variety of visual and verbo-visual media such as painting, movies, blogs, cartoons, and comics, to name a few. Among various modes of autobiographical expressions, graphic medicine took the representation of eating disorder experiences in women one step ahead by offering hitherto underexplored idiosyncratic portrayals of patient experiences.

Graphic medicine, appositely defined as a repertoire of knowledge on phenomenological experience of illnesses, is an artistic as well as an academic discipline that combines subjective experiences and objective representations of disease/disorder/disability conditions. Having emerged from the burgeoning demand for documenting disregarded subjective truths, graphic medicine provides a visual language of self-expression to translate the manifold experiences of suffering. In the conclusion to the *Graphic Medicine Manifesto*, Juliet McMullin states that "graphic medicine is an inspiration" in such a way that it assists individuals in suturing their fragmented selves by offering ways to narrate their illness experiences creatively (Czerwiec 169). While the representation of eating disorders available in popular culture is limited to cathartic and clinical themes, graphic narratives of eating disorders predominantly by women provide a unique articulation of diverse cultural and profoundly feminine experiences that are interlinked with the onset and prognosis of the disorder.

Although many verbal narratives of eating disorders in women have emerged since 1978, not many could transcend the philanthropic and cathartic imperatives of autobiographical writing. However, the visual memoirs taken for this research affirms that graphic medicine enables sufferers to visualize and articulate their subjective experiences of troubles associated with eating disorders. The present study has taken seven well-received graphic narratives on eating disorders. They are Nadia Shivack's *Inside Out: Portrait of an Eating Disorder* (2007), Carol Lay's *The Big Skinny: How I Changed My Fattitude* (2008), Lesley Fairfield's *Tyranny* (2009), Ludovic Debeurme's *Lucille* (2011), Karrie Fransman's *The House That Groaned* (2012), Katie Green's *Lighter Than My Shadow* (2013), and Lacy J. Davis and Jim Kettner's (2016) *Ink in Water: An Illustrated Memoir (Or, How I Kicked Anorexia's Ass and Embraced Body Positivity)*. The select graphic narratives on eating disorders are visual attestations of the fact that eating disorders are caused by a plethora of factors and not merely because women are weak-willed and are obsessed with the concept of thinness perpetuated by the fashion and beauty industries. These graphic pathographies offer new ways of understanding eating disorder experiences from various objective and subjective perspectives. Besides helping the female community of sufferers to understand their experiential realities, these fictional as well as non-fictional graphic narratives also alert the patriarchal society and medical community about the subjective travails of eating disorder sufferers.

These graphic medicine narratives that are mostly written from the sufferer's perspective have pushed eating disorder studies beyond the precincts of biological and cultural research through their unique visual references to the impact of certain feminine experiences such as menstruation. By providing detail oriented description of menarche as an utterly disempowering experience that causes abjection and body image distortion, graphic pathographers such as Green and Fairfield have broadened the vistas of eating disorder research. While the negative impact of body shaming and sexual abuse have been subjects of exhaustive research for a long time, the present study has attempted to understand the contributory role of abjection caused by menstruation and body shaming in women's anorexia. A detailed exploration of the association between abjection and anorexia in the selected graphic pathographies using the theoretical insights of Warin is one of the distinctive features of this book. Thus, the present study underscores how graphic medicine humanizes illness conditions and offers a unique ingress into women's phenomenological experience of eating disorders.

The theoretical spine of this research is the biocultural model which offers a productive understanding of the integration of objective medical knowledge and subjective experiences of an illness. Biocultural research analyses the relationship between culture, health, and healing and does not fail to factor in the popular cultural views of illness as well as the traditional views of biomedical healing. Assimilating a plethora of cultural and biological factors, the biocultural model challenges the reductionistic approach of the biomedical and cultural models. Using the biocultural model, this research investigates how graphic pathographies delineate a unique perspective about eating disorders in women as an experience of abjection, trauma, and powerlessness. In so doing, a holistic and composite understanding of the etiology and implications of eating disorders in women is made possible using graphic medicine narratives. Apart from the biocultures theory, various theoretical strains from trauma studies, comics studies, body studies, feminism, and embodiment are deployed in this research. Consequently, this research has a literary dimension, since it is predicated on certain non-medical themes, such as the role of culture, familial coercion, body shaming, *thinspiration*, abjection, and verbo-visual metaphors. In essence, by applying the biocultural theory on select graphic autobiographical narratives on eating disorders, this book locates eating disorders at the crossroads of culture and biology.

Further, this book is also an affirmation of the potencies of the comics medium that aid disempowered sufferers in depicting their otherwise indescribable experiences during the course of their eating disorders. Accordingly, an attempt is made to present comics as an ingenious artistic medium that is powerful enough to address and process subjective experiential realities of eating disorders. In the analysis of the expressivity of the comics medium, it is found that the use of metaphors aid traumatized sufferers in revisiting and externalizing their experiences, thereby creating artistic ways of self-restoration. While allowing women to document their personal experiences of coercion at multiple levels, the comics medium also aids in foregrounding their victimization and helplessness. Formal affordances such as spatio-temporality, gestures, and economy of the comics medium empower sufferers in articulating their complex sufferings and in depicting the tacit aspects of their chaotic emotions and experiences. In a similar vein, certain structural features of the medium, such as gutter, panels, and non-linearity, underscores that an inherently fragmented medium like comics is a suitable medium to adequately express the fragmentary nature of traumatic experiences. Deploying the verbo-visual strength of the comics medium, female graphic pathographers are creating bold and genuine portrayals of eating disorders that challenge the popular notion that anorexia is a result of the thinspiration fad. For instance, Katie from *Lighter Than My Shadow* illustrates anorexia as a result of familial coercion and sexual abuse. Similarly, Janet in *The House That Groaned* demonstrates the occurrence of anorexia as a result of marital trauma. Some of the other notable characters are Lacy and Lucille who suffer from anorexia caused by various other sociocultural and biocultural factors. Since comics also provide a unique space to restore the disrupted selves of women suffering from eating disorders, the present study reiterates that graphic medicine offers a holistic understanding of eating disorders in females through the comics medium. Thus, after an in-depth analysis of the power of comics in narrating disrupted emotional truths, it is clear that graphic medicine empowers women in communicating disintegrated experiences. In that way, this work is also an attestation of how graphic pathographers are creators of "new visual styles of suffering and illness" who are "subtly altering the discourse of health and the social mediation of illness outside of the clinic" (Czerwiec 118).

Deploying the biocultures framework, this study has analyzed the deleterious impact of certain causative factors, such as familial coercion, body shaming, sexual abuse, and abjection, on women and girls. Although there are plenty of references about insufferable self-repulsion in various anorexia narratives, the concept of abjection has never been deployed to study the etiology of eating disorders. Warin's new-fangled perspectives on anorexia and abjection have strengthened this chapter in its attempt to redefine the intense self-disgust as an instance of abjection by closely reading *Lighter Than My Shadow, Lucille, Inside Out, Tyranny,* and

The House That Groaned. It is evident from the analysis that women tend to experience their bodies as abject and contaminated due to various repulsive bodily experiences caused mainly by menstrual blood flow, sexual abuse, and body shaming. The internalization of the false belief that they are impure affects their self-esteem and confidence in their body. As a result of an increased sense of shame and self-disgust, women would resort to starvation as a punishment or a corrective measure, eventually leading to the rise of eating disorders. While the existing literature on eating disorders repeatedly addresses certain cultural or clinical aspects, graphic medicine is drawing the reader's attention to a condition where abjection instigated by bodily transformations during puberty or a deeply feminine experience of menstruation could also lead to eating disorders.

In an article on demedicalizing anorexia, O'Connor and Esterik emphasize the pressing need for reconfiguring the popular understanding of anorexia by saying that the prevalent discourse on anorexia is "detach[ed] from the anorexic's experiences and values. No wonder treatment programmes are so unsuccessful" (7). Although O'Connor and Esterik criticize biomedicine, they do not deny the fact that anorexics need medical help. But

> medicalizing anorexics and pathologizing their asceticism and other cultural practices have a miserable record of repeated failure. Today, over 130 years after physicians first isolated self-starvation as a disease, biomedicine can neither adequately explain nor reliably cure, nor even rigorously define anorexia. (9)

While this is the case with all popular explanatory models of eating disorders, a biocultural approach that would "put the person back in context" is essential to understand the underlying medical/cultural/psychological causes of eating disorders (9). As O'Connor and Esterik maintain,

> [a]norexics are not culturally but bioculturally constructed. To starve oneself draws on capacities and inclinations that develop only over years. From conception to adolescence, each person's initially wide possibilities progressively narrow as the organism grows and adapts to a particular environment. Day by day, the interaction of biology, culture and chance fix points that shape later interactions, and bit by bit the guiding force of this bio cultural hybrid - a constitution – grows. (8)

Invariably, only a comprehensive theoretical explanation can address various causes or triggers like abjection that have escaped the clinical or cultural scrutiny. Therefore, after close reading various instances of cultural coercion, body image distortion, and abjection in select graphic narratives on eating disorders through the biocultural lens, this book concludes that female graphic pathographers are equipped to add layers to the diverse biocultural meanings of women's starvation using the comics medium. By bravely sharing the subjective elucidations of their eating disorders from both clinical and cultural perspectives, graphic medicine is facilitating the much-needed reconfiguration of the popular understanding of eating disorders as mere psychological problems. Though this book might sound anti-medical at the level of language, it is not in the objectives of the authors to criticize or belittle the accomplishments of medical science in the field of eating disorders. While most of the existing research favors either the biomedical or cultural model of illness, this study is an attempt to understand the infinite potential of graphic medicine to shed light on various underexplored causes and provide a holistic phenomenological understanding of eating disorders in women using the biocultural explanatory model. As Warin notes in the Preface of *Abject Relations*, there are growing calls for "anorexia to be demedicalized and placed within a biocultural context" and this book is an attempt to "respond to these calls by providing an alternative understanding of anorexia" and other eating disorders using graphic medicine (x).

Works Cited

Warin, Megan. *Abject Relations: Everyday Worlds of Anorexia*. Rutgers UP, 2009.
Williams, Ian. "Comics and the Iconography of Illness." *Graphic Medicine Manifesto*, edited Czerwiec MK et al., Penn State UP, 2015, pp. 115–142.

Acknowledgments

I owe a special debt of gratitude to Professor Gurumurthy Neelakantan, Indian Institute of Technology, Kanpur, for teaching me the art of research writing. I would like to thank Jennifer Abbott and Mitchell Manners for their utmost professionalism, enthusiasm, and patient response to numerous questions during the preparation of the manuscript. Special thanks are due to the faculty of the Department of Humanities and Social Sciences, National Institute of Technology (NIT), Tiruchirappalli. Thanks also to the publishers who allowed to reproduce essays contained in this book. Many thanks to my PhD graduate students. The book has immensely benefitted from their conversations, seminars, and class presentations over many years. Dedicated to my wife, Pavithra Ayyapan, and my son, Taran Sathyaraj.

Sathyaraj Venkatesan

I am thankful to my research supervisor, Dr. Sathyaraj Venkatesan, for taking me beyond the immediate boundaries of English literature to the thrilling realm of medical humanities. Heartfelt gratitude to Jennifer Abbot for believing in the possibilities of this work and giving it a place in Routledge. Thanks are also due to the editorial and production teams of Routledge, especially Mitchell Manners for his assistance and patience. For their astonishing generosity and expert comments, I thank M. K. Czerwiec, Mathew Noe, Dr. A. David Lewis, and Katie Green. Many thanks to the librarians of the Cecil Green Library, University of Stanford, California, and Bodleian Library, University of Oxford, for helping me get hold of some neoteric secondary resources.

I am profoundly grateful to Senthil, Raghavi, Aneesh, and Aiswarya for their love. Most of all, I am thankful to my parents for their unconditional support and forbearance. Much love to John, Annu, Mathews, and Rose for the good cheer; and Crystal baby for spreading a glint of hopeful sweetness in my life during times of bleakness.

Earlier versions of chapters 1, 4, and 5 were published as "Towards a Theory of Graphic Medicine" in *Rupkatha Journal on Interdisciplinary Studies in Humanities* (2019); "Feminine Famishment: Graphic Medicine and Anorexia Nervosa" in *Health: An International Journal for Social Study of Health, Illness and Medicine* (2018); and "Anorexia through Creative Metaphors: Women Pathographers and Graphic Medicine" in the *Journal of Graphic Novels and Comics* (2019).

This book is dedicated to my family and friends who were my hope during the inception, evolution, and publication of this work through 2015–2020.

Anu Mary Peter

Index

abjection 6, 92, 95, 100, 102, 103; anorexia 79–82, 101; disgust 88; *Lighter Than My Shadow* 82–87; origin and definitions 77–78; sexual violence to 75; in *Tyranny* 87–90

Abject Relations: Everyday Worlds of Anorexia (Warin) 80, 81, 90–94, 103

Abortion Eve (Farmer and Chevli) 12

aerobic exercise 35; *see also* healthcare

"A History of Scientific English" (Andrews) 8

Andrews, Edmund: "A History of Scientific English" 8

anorexia 2, 18–22, 24, 98; abjection and 79–82; biocultural approach 36–38; biocultural view of 51–52; biomedical identification of 17; body shaming and 43–47; discourses 75; familial pressure 38–43; medical rationalizations of 52; metaphors 60; teenage phase 67

anorexia mirabilis 18, 19

anorexia narratives 101; relationship metaphors in 64–66

anorexia nervosa *see* anorexia

Arya, Rina 79

"At That Time, Nobody Considered It" 38–43

autobiographies: comics 12, 71; on eating disorders 3–4; graphic narratives 12, 56, 82

Barber, Hugh 9

Barry, Lynda 12

Bataille, Georges 78

The Bath of Venus (Boucher) 36

Beatens, Jan 87, 88

A Beautiful Mind (Ron Howard) 10

Bechdel, Alison 12

Bell, Rudolph: *Holy Anorexia* 18–19

Bemporad, Jules R. 37

Benning, Tony B. 25–26

Berger, James 70

Berr, Keith 10

The Big Skinny: How I Changed My Fattitude (Lay) 4

binge eating disorder 23, 38, 61, 62, 93; teenage phase of 67

Binky Brown Meets the Holy Virgin Mary (Green) 3

biocultural approach 27, 29, 76–77; anorexia nervosa 36–38

biocultural model 2, 25–26, 30, 100

biocultural theory 1, 26, 100

biocultures 2–3; framework 101; graphic medicine and 29; research 26, 100

Biocultures Manifesto 27

biological anthropology 26

biomedical model 2, 24, 26, 30; of health and disease 23; limitations of 25

biopsychosocial model of illness 2, 5

body dissatisfaction 44, 47

body image 43–44, 62, 75

body shaming 67, 75, 83, 85–87, 91–95; and anorexia 43–47; negative impact of 100

Bordo, Susan 5, 33, 75; *Unbearable Weight* 37
Boucher, François 36
Brabner, Joyce: *Our Cancer Year* 3
Bray, Abigail 45–46
Brian, Josephine 76
Bright, Susie 12
Brown, Laura S. 75
Brown, Marvelyn: *The Naked Truth* 10
Bruch, Hilde: *The Golden Cage: The Enigma of Anorexia Nervosa* 98
Brumberg, Joan Jacob 5, 17, 20, 24
Bulik, Cynthia 1
bulimia nervosa 22, 23

Carpenter, Karen 21
Charon, Rita 9–10
Chernin, Kim 75
Chevli, Lyn: *Abortion Eve* 12
Chute, Hilary 12
comics 2–3, 15, 46, 71;
    healthcare 13; metaphors, and externalization 57–58; structural features 11; verbo-visual dynamics 65; women and counterculture 12–13
comics medium 3–6, 8, 12, 13, 15, 83, 101; healthcare 11; power 68–70
counterculture 12–13
Court, John P. M. 20; *The Disjointed Historical Trajectory of Anorexia Nervosa Before 1970* 18
creative metaphors 6, 56, 59, 71
Crumb, Aline Kominsky: "Goldie: A Neurotic Woman" 12
Crumb, Sophie 12
cultural association 37; between comics and healthcare 13
cultural construct 17; ideal female body as 34–36
culture 24; body relationship 34; femininity 33; productive yoking 26; role in development of eating disorders 17; in science 26–28
culture-bound syndrome 37
Cushing, Harvey 11
Czerwiec, M. K. 3

Davis, Lacy J.: *Ink in Water: An Illustrated Memoir* 47; *Ink in Water: An Illustrated Memoir (Or, How I Kicked Anorexia's Ass and Embraced Body Positivity)* 4–5
Davis, Lennard J. 2, 5, 17, 26, 27, 30, 37
Davison, Al: *The Spiral Cage* 3
Debeurme, Ludovic: *Lucille* 4, 75, 89
Del Rio, Dolores 35
Denza, Diana 91
Diagnostic and Statistical Manual of Mental Disorders – IV Revised (DSM-R) 21
diet manuals 49, 50
disease: biomedical model of 23; wasting disease 21; *see also* illness
disgust 79, 82, 88, 90–94
The Disjointed Historical Trajectory of Anorexia Nervosa Before 1970 (Court and Kaplan) 18
'Doctors' Failings on Eating Disorders are Costing Lives' (Davies) 1
Douglas, Mary 88; *Purity and Danger* 34
Downie, Robin 9
Dukes, Richard L. 51

eating disorders 1, 2–3, 60, 68, 98; anorexia nervosa 22; autobiographical graphic narratives on 56; binge eating and EDNOS 23; bulimia nervosa 22; clinical explanation of 24; cultural causes of 17; cultural history 18; development in women 17; feminist cultural theorists 76; feminist perspectives 76–78; gendered analyses of 95; graphic medical narratives 33; graphic narratives 99; intricacies 70; literary autobiographies 3; medical boundaries 29; medical introduction 21–23; metaphor 61; pitfalls in models 23–25; portrayals of 4; into postmodern illnesses 38; psychological

explanation of 76; representation of 99; societal norms in etiology of 75; verbal narratives of 99
EDNOS 23
Eisner, Will 83
Engel, George 2, 25, 30
Esterik, P. Van 30, 102
externalization 6, 15, 57–58, 60

Fairfield, Lesley 100; *Tyranny* 4, 6, 33, 48–52, 56, 60–64, 66, 68–70, 76, 87–90
familial pressure 38–43
Farmer, Joyce: *Abortion Eve* 12
'fasting girl' 20
fasting saints 18–19
feminine *see* femininity
feminine beauty 34–36, 48, 51, 86
femininity 21, 51; construct 34; cultural standards 46; culture and 33; standards 67
'Flashes of Hope' 10
Folkman, Susan 77
Fonda, Jane 35
formal affordances 70, 71, 101
Forney, Ellen 12
Foucault, Michael 20
Frank, Arthur 38
Fransman, Karrie: *The House That Groaned* 4, 76, 89–90
Frost, Samantha 27

gender: analyses of eating disorders 95; culture 44, 52; socio-cultural construction 24
Genette, Gerard 39
Gentileschi, Artemisia 36
Giordano, Simona 43
The Golden Cage: The Enigma of Anorexia Nervosa (Bruch) 98
"Goldie: A Neurotic Woman" (Crumb) 12
Goldner-Vukov, Mila 93
Gordon, Richard 37
graphic medical narratives 65, 71
graphic medicine 2–5, 8, 15, 71, 98, 99, 102, 103; biocultures 29; definition and scope 13–14; iconography of illness 59–60
Graphic Medicine Manifesto 13, 99

graphic medicine narratives 3–4, 14, 15, 95, 99, 100
graphic pathographers 6, 56, 58, 60, 99–101, 103
graphic pathographies 3, 14, 29, 75, 99, 100
Green, Justin: *Binky Brown Meets the Holy Virgin Mary* 3
Green, Katie 100; *Lighter Than My Shadow* 4, 6, 33, 50–52, 56, 60, 66–68, 76, 82–87, 91–94 (*see also Lighter Than My Shadow* (Green))
Green, Michael J. 3
Groensteen, Thierry 68
Grozs, Elizabeth 84
The Guardian 1
guilt 40–41
Gull, William Withey 21, 22

Hansen, Bert: "Medical History for the Masses: How American Comic Books Celebrated Heroes of Medicine in the 1940s" 11
Harcourt, Diana 47
healthcare: biomedical model 23; comics and 13; comics medium 11
health humanities 8, 14, 15
Hepburn, Katherine 35
Hepworth, Julie: *The Social Construction of Anorexia Nervosa* 19
Holy Anorexia (Bell) 18–19
Horton, Scott L. 68
The House That Groaned (Fransman) 4, 6, 76, 89–90
Howard, Ron: *A Beautiful Mind* 10
Huang, Michelle N. 67
Hudson, James I. 37
humanization, of medical science 8–9
hysteria 19–21

ideal female body 15, 19, 88; contemporary notions 33; cultural constructs 34–36, 44–45; cultural representation 3; evolution 34; *see also* women
illness: across media, representation 10–11; iconography 59–60;

mental and physical 21; ordeals
9–10; phenomenology 98
*Illness and Culture in the
Postmodern Age* (Morris) 38
*Ink in Water: An Illustrated Memoir
(Or, How I Kicked Anorexia's Ass
and Embraced Body Positivity)*
(Davis and Kettner) 4–5, 47
*Inside Out: Portrait of an Eating
Disorder* (Shivack) 4, 6, 56, 60,
64–66, 75–76, 89, 90
It Ain't Me Babe 12

Johnson, Mark 57

Kahlo, Frida: *The Wounded
Deer* 10
Kaplan, Allan S. 20; *The Disjointed
Historical Trajectory of Anorexia
Nervosa Before 1970* 18
Krauss, Rosalind 15
Kristeva, Julia 37, 78, 79, 81;
concept of abjection 80, 82, 85
Kruif, Paul de 11

Lakoff, George 56, 57
Lay, Carol: *The Big Skinny: How I
Changed My Fattitude* 4
Lazarus, Richard S. 77
Levack, Brian P.: *The Witch-Hunt in
Early Modern Europe* 19
Lorch, Barbara Day 51
Lovato, Demi 10
Lucille (Debeurme) 4, 6, 75, 89
Lupton, Deborah 47

Martin, Emily: *The Woman in the
Body* 81
McCloud, Scott 40
McMullin, Juliet 99
media 60; representation of illness
10–11; thinspiration 47–51
medical comics 11
"Medical History for the Masses:
How American Comic Books
Celebrated Heroes of Medicine in
the 1940s" (Hansen) 11
medical humanities 8–9
medical science 11, 24, 29, 37, 76;
to accept anorexia nervosa as
illness 98; biocultural approach

27; in eating disorders field 103;
humanization 8–9
medicine: comics 2, 8; science 8; *see
also* graphic medicine; narrative
medicine
Mendes, Willy 12
Menninghaus, Winfried 90
menstrual blood 81, 84, 85
menstruation 81–82, 99, 100; in
Lighter Than My Shadow 82–87;
in *Tyranny* 87–90
metaphors 56–58, 100–101;
of anorexia 60; in anorexia
narratives, relationship 64–66;
eating disorders 61; illness
narratives 59; of pervasiveness
66–68; of self-oppression 60–64
Michelangelo: *La Pieta* 10
Middle Ages 18–19, 29
Millman, Marcia 75
miracle maidens 18–19
Monroe, Marilyn 35
Morris, David 33; *Illness and
Culture in the Postmodern Age* 38
Morris, David B. 5, 17, 26, 27, 30, 37
Morton, Richard 21;
*Phthisiologia, Or, A Treatise of
Consumptions* 98
Mulholland, Matthew J. 71
Myers, Kimberly R. 3

The Naked Truth (Brown) 10
Napier, A. David 27
narrative medicine 8–10, 13, 14
"Neil! You Look Like a Man!" 43–47

O'Connor, Richard A. 30, 102
Our Cancer Year (Pekar and
Brabner) 3

paintings 36; *La Pieta* 10; *The
Wounded Deer* 10
Pasteur, Louis 11
Pekar, Harvey: *Our Cancer Year* 3
Petty, Amber 35
phenomenology: of eating disorders
29, 75, 100, 103; female anorexics
79, 80; illnesses 98
*Phthisiologia, Or, A Treatise of
Consumptions* (Morton) 98
physical assault 92, 93

Pope Jr, Harrison G. 37
postmodern illnesses 38
post-structuralism 77
Powers of Horror 78
psychological troubles 56
puberty 6, 48, 82, 102
public space 84
punishment 42–43, 102
Purity and Danger (Douglas) 34

Rebraca, Louise: *Shives* 18
Reed, Walter 11
Refaie, Elizabeth El 5, 6, 56, 58, 59, 61
relationship metaphors, in anorexia narratives 64–66
Robbins, Trina 12
Rumsey, Nichola 47
Russell, Gerard 22

Sarton, George 8, 27
Satrapi, Marjane 12
Scarry, Elaine 57
self-destructive behavior 56
self-disgust 85, 87, 89–94, 101, 102
self-esteem 33, 36, 40, 41, 44, 45, 64, 82, 89–91, 102
self-expression 11, 58, 98–99
self-oppression, metaphor 60–64
self-realization 89
self-restoration 71, 101
self-starvation 18–21, 29, 77, 95, 98
sexual abuse 75, 81, 101; negative impact 100; self-disgust 90–94
Shivack, Nadia: *Inside Out: Portrait of an Eating Disorder* 4, 6, 56, 60, 64–66, 75–76, 89, 90
Showalter, Elaine 20
size zero figure 35
slenderness 33, 38, 48, 51, 62, 89
Smith, Scott T. 3
social abjection 78, 81
The Social Construction of Anorexia Nervosa (Hepworth) 19
social/cultural anthropology 26
socio-cultural construct 34; of gender 24
socio-cultural rigidities 33
Sontag, Susan 59
The Spiral Cage (Davison) 3
Squier, Susan M. 3, 13, 43

starvation 5, 18–21, 44, 47, 62, 75, 88, 102, 103
suffering, spectacles of 10–11
"symbol of society" 34

thinspiration 47–51, 100, 101
Thompson, Becky 77
Tits 'n' Clits Comix 12
traditional biomedical approach 25
True Comics 11
Tyler, Imogen 81
Tyranny (Fairfield) 4, 6, 33, 48–52, 56, 60–64, 66, 68–70, 76; menstruation and abjection in 87–90

Unbearable Weight (Bordo) 37

verbal expressions 56, 71
verbo-visual metaphors 6, 40, 52, 58, 59, 65, 70, 71, 100, 101
visual metaphor 46, 58, 67, 68, 70, 71, 92
vulnerability 13, 41, 43, 51

Walsh, Karen 91
Warin, Megan 5, 64, 75, 76, 78, 79–82, 100; *Abject Relations: Everyday Worlds of Anorexia* 80, 81, 90–94
wasting disease 21
Waugh, Patricia 27, 28
Wegner, Gesine 3
Western Christianity 18
Williams, Ian 3, 6, 13, 56, 60, 67, 69
Wilson, Susannah 60–61
Wimmin's Comix 12
The Witch-Hunt in Early Modern Europe (Levack) 19
Wolf, Naomi 36
The Woman in the Body (Martin) 81
women: counterculture and comics 12–13; diet of 51; eating disorders development 17; menstruation and body shaming 100; psychological explanation of eating disorders 76; starvation 19–21, 75; Western Christianity 18; *see also* ideal female body
The Wounded Deer (Kahlo) 10

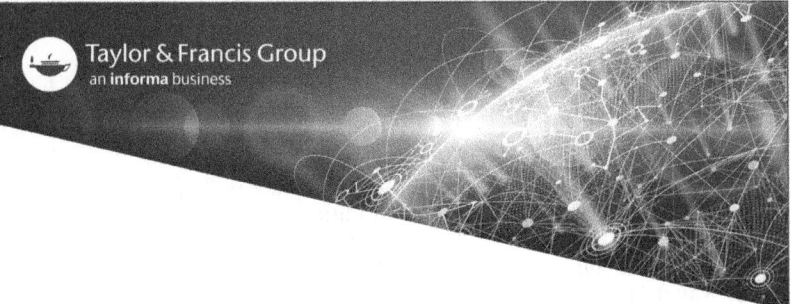

Taylor & Francis eBooks

www.taylorfrancis.com

A single destination for eBooks from Taylor & Francis
with increased functionality and an improved user
experience to meet the needs of our customers.

90,000+ eBooks of award-winning academic content in
Humanities, Social Science, Science, Technology, Engineering,
and Medical written by a global network of editors and authors.

TAYLOR & FRANCIS EBOOKS OFFERS:

A streamlined
experience for
our library
customers

A single point
of discovery
for all of our
eBook content

Improved
search and
discovery of
content at both
book and
chapter level

REQUEST A FREE TRIAL
support@taylorfrancis.com

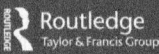
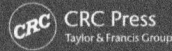